CHILDREN AND SECONDHAND SMOKE EXPOSURE

CHILDREN AND SECONDHAND SMOKE EXPOSURE

JANICE R. HARRINGTON
EDITOR

Nova Science Publishers, Inc.
New York

Copyright © 2009 by Nova Science Publishers, Inc.

All rights reserved. No part of this book may be reproduced, stored in a retrieval system or transmitted in any form or by any means: electronic, electrostatic, magnetic, tape, mechanical photocopying, recording or otherwise without the written permission of the Publisher.

For permission to use material from this book please contact us:
Telephone 631-231-7269; Fax 631-231-8175
Web Site: http://www.novapublishers.com

NOTICE TO THE READER
The Publisher has taken reasonable care in the preparation of this book, but makes no expressed or implied warranty of any kind and assumes no responsibility for any errors or omissions. No liability is assumed for incidental or consequential damages in connection with or arising out of information contained in this book. The Publisher shall not be liable for any special, consequential, or exemplary damages resulting, in whole or in part, from the readers' use of, or reliance upon, this material.

Independent verification should be sought for any data, advice or recommendations contained in this book. In addition, no responsibility is assumed by the publisher for any injury and/or damage to persons or property arising from any methods, products, instructions, ideas or otherwise contained in this publication.

This publication is designed to provide accurate and authoritative information with regard to the subject matter covered herein. It is sold with the clear understanding that the Publisher is not engaged in rendering legal or any other professional services. If legal or any other expert assistance is required, the services of a competent person should be sought. FROM A DECLARATION OF PARTICIPANTS JOINTLY ADOPTED BY A COMMITTEE OF THE AMERICAN BAR ASSOCIATION AND A COMMITTEE OF PUBLISHERS.

LIBRARY OF CONGRESS CATALOGING-IN-PUBLICATION DATA
Available upon request
ISBN: 978-1-60692-587-4

Published by Nova Science Publishers, Inc. ✦ New York

CONTENTS

Preface		vii
Foreword		1
Introduction		3
Chapter 1	Excerpts from Chapter 1. Introduction, Summary, and Conclusions	5
Chapter 2	Excerpts from Chapter 4. Prevalence of Exposure to Secondhand Smoke	15
Chapter 3	Excerpts from Chapter 5. Reproductive and Developmental Effects from Exposure to Secondhand Smoke	45
Chapter 4	Excerpts from Chapter 6. Respiratory Effects in Children from Exposure to Secondhand Smoke	89
Chapter 5	Excerpts from Chapter 10. Control of Secondhand Smoke Exposure	129
Index		157

PREFACE

The first Surgeon General's report to conclude that involuntary exposure of non smokers to secondhand smoke causes disease was published more than 20 years ago. That report concluded that children whose parents smoke are more likely to experience respiratory infections and respiratory symptoms.

Today, massive and conclusive scientific evidence documents the serious health risks that secondhand smoke poses to children, and the list of these health conditions has lengthened. The 2006 Surgeon General's report on *The Health Consequences of Involuntary Exposure to Tobacco Smoke* concludes that children who are exposed to secondhand smoke are at an increased risk for sudden infant death syndrome, lower respiratory infections, middle ear disease, more severe asthma, respiratory symptoms, and slowed lung growth. Because their respiratory, immune, and nervous systems are still developing, children are especially vulnerable to the health effects of secondhand smoke. In addition, young chil dren typically are exposed to secondhand smoke involuntarily and have limited options for avoiding exposure. They depend on their parents and on adults around them for pro tection.

On average, children are exposed to more secondhand smoke than nonsmok ing adults. Most of these children are exposed to secondhand smoke at home. Children continue to be exposed in their homes as a result of the smoking of their parents and other adults. Among children younger than 18 years of age, approximately 22 percent are exposed to secondhand smoke in their homes, with estimates ranging from 11.7 percent in Utah to 34.2 percent in Kentucky.

We know that making homes smoke-free reduces secondhand smoke exposure among children and nonsmoking adults, helps smokers quit, and decreases smoking ini tiation among youth. What we don't know, due to a lack of definitive research in this area, is what interventions are most effective in convincing parents to take this step. Targeted, sustained research in this area is urgently needed, with a special focus on evaluating ongoing initiatives to establish what works.

The evidence suggests that vehicles can also be a significant source of secondhand smoke exposure for children. Children can be regularly exposed to secondhand smoke when parents or other adults smoke in these vehicles while they are present. The concentrations of secondhand smoke in vehicles where smoking is occurring can reach very high levels. Making vehicles smoke-free would be expected to reduce children's secondhand smoke exposure. Again, the challenge is what approaches are effective and appropriate for achieving this objective. To date, it appears that few educational campaigns promoting smoke-free home rules have promoted the adoption of similar rules in vehicles. The U.S. Environmental Protection Agency has recently begun to address this setting in its educational efforts.

Parents want nothing but the best for their children. Many parents make great sacrifices for their children's benefit. If they knew how harmful secondhand smoke was to children, most parents would take steps to protect them. In fact, many parents do attempt to protect their children from secondhand smoke, but take measures that are ineffective, such as smoking by a window or fan, opening a window, or limiting smoking to certain rooms. The 2006 Surgeon General's report makes clear that establishing a completely smoke-free home is the only effective way to eliminate secondhand smoke exposure in this setting. It is important that parents receive this message. Educational efforts can play a crucial role in helping parents understand why they need to protect their children from this health hazard and how to do so effectively.

Pediatricians are especially well-positioned to influence parents on this issue. Because of the high levels of secondhand smoke exposure among young children and the health problems they experience as a result, their exposure should be considered a significant medical issue. Well-child visits provide regular opportunities to screen children for exposure and to educate parents about the importance of protecting children from secondhand smoke. Parents who smoke are likely to see a pediatrician more often than they see their own physicians. Pediatrician visits occasioned by an illness related to secondhand smoke exposure, such as pneumonia, offer a unique teachable moment. Pediatricians can advise parents to quit smoking, and can refer them to the range of evidence-based cessation aids that are available, including cessation assistance through 1-800-QUITNOW and FDA-approved cessation medications. In the interim, pediatricians can encourage parents to make their homes and cars smoke-free and to always go outside to smoke. The evidence indicates that, in addition to protecting their children, this step will also help parents and caregivers to quit.

Exposure to secondhand smoke among children remains a major public health prob lem. Of the more than 126 million U.S. nonsmokers who are still exposed, almost 40 mil lion are children aged 3 to 18 years. We now have clear evidence that only completely smoke-free environments can eliminate secondhand smoke exposure and its related health risks. We need to apply this knowledge to educate parents to take action to make the set tings where their children spend time smoke-free. The public's attitudes and social norms toward secondhand smoke exposure have changed significantly; it's high time that we build on these changes to protect our children.

Kenneth P. Moritsugu,
M.D., M.P.H.
Acting Surgeon General

In: Children and Secondhand Smoke Exposure
Editor: J. R. Harrington

ISBN: 978-1-60692-587-4
© 2009 Nova Science Publishers, Inc.

FOREWORD

The Health Consequences of Involuntary Exposure to Tobacco Smoke provided a progress report on the remarkable reduction in involuntary exposure to secondhand smoke that has been achieved over the last 20 years. It also noted the gaps and disparities that remain in this regard. This excerpt highlights the serious health risks that secondhand smoke expo sure poses to our children and the need to extend the same protections to them that many U.S. adults already enjoy.

Children are more heavily exposed to secondhand smoke than adults. Almost 60 percent of U.S. children aged 3-11 years, or almost 22 million children, are exposed to secondhand smoke. A *Healthy People 2010* objective calls for reducing the proportion of children aged 6 years and younger who are regularly exposed to secondhand smoke in the home from 20 percent in 1998 to 6 percent by 2010. According to the 2005 National Health Interview Survey, this proportion may already be as low as 8 percent, suggesting that, with sustained and expanded efforts, we may be able to achieve this target.

However, too many children continue to be exposed. Children who are exposed to secondhand smoke are at an increased risk for sudden infant death syndrome, lower respiratory infections, middle ear disease, more severe asthma, respiratory symptoms, and slowed lung growth. The California Environmental Protection Agency recently estimated that 430 infants die from sudden infant death syndrome in the United States every year as a result of secondhand smoke exposure. The same agency also estimated that secondhand smoke exposure is responsible for 202,300 asthma episodes and 790,000 doctor appoint ments for U.S. children with ear infections annually. Children whose parents smoke and who grow up in homes where smoking is allowed are also more likely to become smokers themselves.

The home is the major setting where children are exposed. Children who live in homes where smoking is allowed have higher levels of cotinine, a biological marker for secondhand smoke exposure, than children who live in homes where smoking is not allowed. One of the strongest predictors of children's cotinine levels is the number of ciga rettes smoked daily in the home. Almost one in four children aged 3 to 11 years lives in a household with at least one smoker, compared to only about one in fourteen nonsmoking adults. Children are also exposed to secondhand smoke in vehicles.

Low-income children and African American children are disproportionately exposed to secondhand smoke. In fact, cotinine levels suggest that African American children are among the most heavily exposed of any population group. These disparities need to be better understood and addressed.

This excerpt moves forward the mission of CDC to promote and protect Americans' health. I applaud those who have had a part in focusing our national attention on acceler ating our progress in reducing the burden of disease that smoking and secondhand smoke exposure continue to impose on our nation.

Julie Louise Gerberding, M.D., M.P.H.
Director

Centers for Disease Control and Prevention and
Administrator
Agency for Toxic Substances and Disease Registry

INTRODUCTION

These excerpts from the 2006 Surgeon General's report, *The Health Consequences of Involuntary Exposure to Tobacco Smoke,* highlight the harmful effects of secondhand smoke expo sure on children. The text and tables that follow are drawn directly from the report that was released previously by the Surgeon General (USDHHS 2006).

The report concluded that secondhand smoke causes premature death and disease in children. In addition, the report also concluded that children who are exposed to second hand smoke are at an increased risk for sudden infant death syndrome, lower respiratory infections, middle ear disease, more severe asthma, respiratory symptoms, and slowed lung growth. The California Environmental Protection Agency (Cal/EPA) has estimated that 430 infants die from sudden infant death syndrome in the United States every year as a result of secondhand smoke exposure (Cal/EPA 2005). The same report also estimated that second hand smoke exposure is responsible for 202,300 asthma episodes and 790,000 doctor appoint ments for U.S. children with ear infections annually.

Children and teens are more heavily exposed to secondhand smoke than adults. Almost 60 percent of U.S. children aged 3 to 11 years, or almost 22 million children, are exposed to secondhand smoke.

Because their respiratory, immune, and nervous systems are still developing, children are especially vulnerable to the health effects of secondhand smoke. In addition, young chil dren typically are exposed to secondhand smoke involuntarily and have limited options for avoiding exposure. They depend on their parents and on other adults to protect them.

The home is the major setting where children are exposed to secondhand smoke. Chil dren who live in homes where smoking is allowed have higher levels of cotinine, a biological marker for secondhand smoke exposure, than children who live in homes where smoking is not allowed (CDC 2005). Almost one in four children aged 3 to 11 years lives in a household with at least one smoker, compared to only about 7 percent of nonsmoking adults.

The dramatic strides that have been made over the past 20 years in reducing nonsmokers' secondhand smoke exposure has to some extent left children behind. While increasing numbers of homes, including many homes where smokers live, are going smoke-free, the pace of progress in this setting has lagged behind the spread of smoke-free environments in workplaces and public places. It is ironic that the Americans who are at the greatest risk from secondhand smoke and who are least able to defend themselves are also the least protected and the most heavily exposed.

It is high time that we address this disparity. We need to act now to ensure that all parents have the facts they need to make informed decisions to protect their families from this completely preventable health hazard.

REFERENCES

California Environmental Protection Agency. *Proposed Identification of Environmental Tobacco Smoke as a Toxic Air Contaminant. Part B: Health Effects*. Sacramento (CA): California Environmental Protection Agency, Office of Environmental Health Hazard Assessment, 2005.

Centers for Disease Control and Prevention. *Third National Report on Human Exposure to Environmental Chemicals*. Atlanta: U.S. Department of Health and Human Services, Centers for Disease Control and Prevention, National Center for Environmental Health, 2005. NCEH Publication No. 05-0570.

U.S. Department of Health and Human Services. *The Health Consequences of Involuntary Exposure to Tobacco Smoke: A Report of the Surgeon General*. Atlanta: U.S. Department of Health and Human Services, Centers for Disease Control and Prevention, National Center for Chronic Disease Prevention and Health Promotion, Office on Smoking and Health, 2006.

Chapter 1

EXCERPTS FROM CHAPTER 1. INTRODUCTION, SUMMARY, AND CONCLUSIONS

INTRODUCTION

The topic of passive or involuntary smoking was first addressed in the 1972 U.S. Surgeon Gener al's report (*The Health Consequences of Smoking*, U.S. Department of Health, Education, and Welfare [USD HEW] 1972), only eight years after the first Surgeon General's report on the health consequences of active smoking (USDHEW 1964). Surgeon General Dr. Jesse Steinfeld had raised concerns about this topic, lead ing to its inclusion in that report. According to the 1972 report, nonsmokers inhale the mixture of side- stream smoke given off by a smoldering cigarette and mainstream smoke exhaled by a smoker, a mixture now referred to as "secondhand smoke" or "environ mental tobacco smoke." Cited experimental studies showed that smoking in enclosed spaces could lead to high levels of cigarette smoke components in the air. For carbon monoxide (CO) specifically, levels in enclosed spaces could exceed levels then permitted in outdoor air. The studies supported a conclusion that "an atmosphere contaminated with tobacco smoke can contribute to the discomfort of many individuals" (USDHEW 1972, p. 7). The possibility that CO emitted from cigarettes could harm persons with chronic heart or lung disease was also mentioned.

Secondhand tobacco smoke was then addressed in greater depth in Chapter 4 (Involuntary Smoking) of the 1975 Surgeon General's report, *The Health Conse- quences of Smoking* (USDHEW 1975). The chapter noted that involuntary smoking takes place when nonsmok ers inhale both sidestream and exhaled mainstream smoke and that this "smoking" is "involuntary" when "the exposure occurs as an unavoidable consequence of breathing in a smoke-filled environment" (p. 87). The report covered exposures and potential health conse quences of involuntary smoking, and the researchers concluded that smoking on buses and airplanes was annoying to nonsmokers and that involuntary smok ing had potentially adverse consequences for persons with heart and lung diseases. Two studies on nicotine concentrations in nonsmokers raised concerns about nicotine as a contributing factor to atherosclerotic cardiovascular disease in nonsmokers.

The 1979 Surgeon General's report, *Smoking and Health: A Report of the Surgeon General* (USDHEW 1979), also contained a chapter entitled "Involuntary Smoking." The chapter stressed that "attention to involuntary smoking is of recent vintage, and only limited information regarding the health effects of such exposure upon the nonsmoker is available" (p. 11–35). The chapter concluded with recommenda tions for research including epidemiologic and clini cal studies. The 1982 Surgeon General's report specifi cally addressed smoking and cancer (U.S. Department of Health and Human Services [USDHHS] 1982). By 1982, there were three published epidemiologic stud ies on involuntary smoking and lung cancer, and the 1982 Surgeon General's report included a brief chapter on this topic. That chapter commented on the meth odologic difficulties inherent in such studies, includ ing exposure assessment, the lengthy interval during which exposures are likely to be relevant, and account ing for exposures to other carcinogens. Nonetheless, the report concluded that "Although the currently available evidence is not sufficient to conclude that passive or involuntary smoking causes lung cancer in nonsmokers, the evidence does raise concern about a possible serious public health problem" (p. 251).

Involuntary smoking was also reviewed in the 1984 report, which focused on chronic obstructive pulmonary disease and smoking (USDHHS 1984). Chapter 7 (Passive Smoking) of that report included a comprehensive review of the mounting information on smoking by parents and the effects on respiratory health of their children, data on irritation of the eye, and the more limited evidence on pulmonary effects of involuntary smoking on adults. The chapter began with a compilation of measurements of tobacco smoke components in various indoor environments. The extent of the data had increased substantially since 1972. By 1984, the data included measurements of more specific indicators such as acrolein and nicotine, and less specific indicators such as particulate matter (PM), nitrogen oxides, and CO. The report reviewed new evidence on exposures of nonsmokers using biomarkers, with substantial information on levels of cotinine, a major nicotine metabolite. The report anticipated future conclusions with regard to respira tory effects of parental smoking on child respiratory health.

Involuntary smoking was the topic for the entire 1986 Surgeon General's report, *The Health Consequences of Involuntary Smoking* (USDHHS 1986). In its 359 pages, the report covered the full breadth of the topic, addressing toxicology and dosimetry of tobacco smoke; the relevant evidence on active smoking; patterns of exposure of nonsmokers to tobacco smoke; the epidemiologic evidence on involuntary smoking and disease risks for infants, children, and adults; and policies to control involuntary exposure to tobacco smoke. That report concluded that involuntary smoking caused lung cancer in lifetime nonsmoking adults and was associated with adverse effects on respiratory health in children. The report also stated that simply separating smokers and nonsmokers within the same airspace reduced but did not eliminate exposure to secondhand smoke. All of these findings are relevant to public health and public policy. The lung cancer conclusion was based on extensive information already available on the carcinogenicity of active smoking, the qualitative similarities between secondhand and mainstream smoke, the uptake of tobacco smoke components by nonsmokers, and the epidemiologic data on involuntary smoking. The three major conclusions of the report, led Dr. C. Everett Koop, Surgeon General at the time, to comment in his preface that "the right of smokers to smoke ends where their behavior affects the health and well-being of others; furthermore, it is the smokers' responsibility to ensure that they do not expose nonsmokers to the potential [sic] harmful effects of tobacco smoke" (USDHHS 1986, p. xii).

Two other reports published in 1986 also reached the conclusion that involuntary smoking increased the risk for lung cancer. The International Agency for Research on Cancer (IARC) of the World Health Organization concluded that "passive smoking gives rise to some risk of cancer" (IARC 1986, p. 314). In its monograph on tobacco smoking, the agency supported this conclusion on the basis of the characteristics of sidestream and mainstream smoke, the absorption of tobacco smoke materials during an involuntary exposure, and the nature of dose-response relationships for carcinogenesis. In the same year, the National Research Council (NRC) also concluded that involuntary smoking increases the incidence of lung cancer in nonsmokers (NRC 1986). In reaching this conclusion, the NRC report cited the biologic plausibility of the association between exposure to secondhand smoke and lung cancer and the supporting epidemiologic evidence. On the basis of a pooled analysis of the epidemiologic data adjusted for bias, the report concluded that the best estimate for the excess risk of lung cancer in nonsmokers married to smokers was 25 percent, compared with nonsmokers married to nonsmokers. With regard to the effects of involuntary smoking on children, the NRC report commented on the literature linking secondhand smoke exposures from parental smoking to increased risks for respiratory symptoms and infections and to a slightly diminished rate of lung growth.

Since 1986, the conclusions with regard to both the carcinogenicity of secondhand smoke and the adverse effects of parental smoking on the health of children have been echoed and expanded. In 1992, the U.S. Environmental Protection Agency (EPA) published its risk assessment of secondhand smoke as a carcinogen (USEPA 1992). The agency's evaluation drew on toxicologic information on secondhand smoke and the extensive literature on active smoking. A comprehensive meta-analysis of the 31 epidemiologic studies of secondhand smoke and lung cancer published up to that time was central to the decision to classify secondhand smoke as a group A carcinogen—namely, a known human carcinogen. Estimates of approximately 3,000 U.S. lung cancer deaths per year in nonsmokers were attributed to secondhand smoke. The report also covered other respiratory health effects in children and adults and concluded that involuntary smoking is causally associated with several adverse respiratory effects in children. There was also a quantitative risk assessment for the impact of involuntary smoking on childhood asthma and lower respiratory tract infections in young children.

In the decade since the 1992 EPA report, scientific panels continued to evaluate the mounting evidence linking involuntary smoking to adverse health effects. The most recent was the 2005 report of the California Environmental Protection Agency (Cal/EPA 2005). Over time, research has repeatedly affirmed the conclusions of the 1986 Surgeon General's report and studies have further identified causal associations of involuntary smoking with diseases and other health disorders. The epidemiologic evidence on involuntary smoking has markedly expanded since 1986, as have the data on exposure to tobacco smoke in the many environments where people spend time. An understanding of the mechanisms by which involuntary smoking causes disease has also deepened.

As part of the environmental health hazard assessment, Cal/EPA identified specific health effects causally associated with exposure to secondhand smoke. The agency estimated the annual excess deaths in the United States that are attributable to secondhand smoke exposure for specific disorders: sudden infant death syndrome (SIDS), cardiac-related illnesses (ischemic heart disease), and lung cancer (Cal/EPA 2005). For the excess incidence of other health outcomes, either new estimates were provided or estimates from the 1997 health hazard assessment were used without any revisions (Cal/EPA 1997). Overall, Cal/EPA estimated that about 50,000 excess deaths result annually from exposure to secondhand smoke (Cal/EPA 2005). Estimated annual excess deaths for the total U.S. population are about 3,400 (a range of 3,423 to 8,866) from lung cancer, 46,000 (a range of 22,700 to

69,600) from cardiac-related illnesses, and 430 from SIDS. The agency also estimated that between 24,300 and 71,900 low birth weight or preterm deliveries, about 202,300 episodes of childhood asthma (new cases and exacer bations), between 150,000 and 300,000 cases of lower respiratory illness in children, and about 789,700 cases of middle ear infections in children occur each year in the United States as a result of exposure to second hand smoke.

This new 2006 Surgeon General's report returns to the topic of involuntary smoking. The health effects of involuntary smoking have not received compre hensive coverage in this series of reports since 1986. Reports since then have touched on selected aspects of the topic: the 1994 report on tobacco use among young people (USDHHS 1994), the 1998 report on tobacco use among U.S. racial and ethnic minorities (USDHHS 1998), and the 2001 report on women and smoking (USDHHS 2001). As involuntary smoking remains widespread in the United States and else where, the preparation of this report was motivated by the persistence of involuntary smoking as a public health problem and the need to evaluate the substan tial new evidence reported since 1986. This report sub stantially expands the list of topics that were included in the 1986 report. Additional topics include SIDS, developmental effects, and other reproductive effects; heart disease in adults; and cancer sites beyond the lung. For some associations of involuntary smoking with adverse health effects, only a few studies were reviewed in 1986 (e.g., ear disease in children); now, the relevant literature is substantial. Consequently, this report uses meta-analysis to quantitatively summa rize evidence as appropriate. Following the approach used in the 2004 report (*The Health Consequences of Smoking*, USDHHS 2004), this 2006 report also system atically evaluates the evidence for causality, judging the extent of the evidence available and then making an inference as to the nature of the association.

DEFINITIONS AND TERMINOLOGY

The inhalation of tobacco smoke by nonsmokers has been variably referred to as "passive smoking" or "involuntary smoking." Smokers, of course, also inhale secondhand smoke. Cigarette smoke contains both particles and gases generated by the combustion at high temperatures of tobacco, paper, and addi tives. The smoke inhaled by nonsmokers that con taminates indoor spaces and outdoor environments has often been referred to as "secondhand smoke" or "environmental tobacco smoke." This inhaled smoke is the mixture of sidestream smoke released by the smoldering cigarette and the mainstream smoke that is exhaled by a smoker. Sidestream smoke, generated at lower temperatures and under somewhat different combustion conditions than mainstream smoke, tends to have higher concentrations of many of the toxins found in cigarette smoke (USDHHS 1986). However, it is rapidly diluted as it travels away from the burning cigarette.

Secondhand smoke is an inherently dynamic mixture that changes in characteristics and concentration with the time since it was formed and the distance it has traveled. The smoke particles change in size and composition as gaseous components are volatilized and moisture content changes; gaseous elements of secondhand smoke may be adsorbed onto materials, and particle concentrations drop with both dilution in the air or environment and impaction on surfaces, including the lungs or on the body. Because of its dynamic nature, a specific quantitative definition of secondhand smoke cannot be offered.

This report uses the term secondhand smoke in preference to environmental tobacco smoke, even though the latter may have been used more frequently in previous reports. The descriptor "secondhand" captures the involuntary nature of the exposure, while "environmental" does not. This report also refers to the inhalation of secondhand smoke as involuntary smoking, acknowledging that most nonsmokers do not want to inhale tobacco smoke. The exposure of the fetus to tobacco smoke, whether from active smoking by the mother or from her exposure to secondhand smoke, also constitutes involuntary smoking.

Major Conclusions

This report returns to involuntary smoking, the topic of the 1986 Surgeon General's report. Since then, there have been many advances in the research on secondhand smoke, and substantial evidence has been reported over the ensuing 20 years. This report uses the revised language for causal conclusions that was implemented in the 2004 Surgeon General's report (USDHHS 2004). Each chapter provides a comprehensive review of the evidence, a quantitative synthesis of the evidence if appropriate, and a rigorous assessment of sources of bias that may affect interpretations of the findings. The reviews in this report reaffirm and strengthen the findings of the 1986 report. With regard to the involuntary exposure of nonsmokers to tobacco smoke, the scientific evidence now supports the following major conclusions:

The following conclusions are supported by text in the full report that may not be included in this excerpt. The full report can be accessed at http://www.surgeongeneral.gov/library/secondhandsmoke/report/.

1. Secondhand smoke causes premature death and disease in children and in adults who do not smoke.
2. Children exposed to secondhand smoke are at an increased risk for sudden infant death syndrome (SIDS), acute respiratory infections, ear problems, and more severe asthma. Smoking by parents causes respiratory symptoms and slows lung growth in their children.
3. Exposure of adults to secondhand smoke has immediate adverse effects on the cardiovascular system and causes coronary heart disease and lung cancer.
4. The scientific evidence indicates that there is no risk-free level of exposure to secondhand smoke.
5. Many millions of Americans, both children and adults, are still exposed to secondhand smoke in their homes and workplaces despite substantial progress in tobacco control.
6. Eliminating smoking in indoor spaces fully pro tects nonsmokers from exposure to secondhand smoke. Separating smokers from nonsmokers, cleaning the air, and ventilating buildings cannot eliminate exposures of nonsmokers to second hand smoke.

REFERENCES

California Environmental Protection Agency. *Health Effects of Exposure to Environmental Tobacco Smoke.* Sacramento (CA): California Environmental Pro tection Agency, Office of Environmental Health Hazard Assessment, Reproductive and Cancer Hazard Assessment Section and Air Toxicology and Epidemiology Section, 1997.

California Environmental Protection Agency. *Proposed Identification of Environmental Tobacco Smoke as a Toxic Air Contaminant. Part B: Health Effects.* Sacra mento (CA): California Environmental Protection Agency, Office of Environmental Health Hazard Assessment, 2005.

International Agency for Research on Cancer. *IARC Monographs on the Evaluation of the Carcinogenic Risk of Chemicals to Humans: Tobacco Smoking.* Vol. 38. Lyon (France): International Agency for Research on Cancer, 1986.

National Research Council. *Environmental Tobacco Smoke: Measuring Exposures and Assessing Health Effects.* Washington: National Academy Press, 1986.

U.S. Department of Health and Human Services. *The Health Consequences of Smoking: Cancer. A Report of the Surgeon General.* Rockville (MD): U.S. Depart ment of Health and Human Services, Public Health Service, Office on Smoking and Health. 1982. DHHS Publication No. (PHS) 82-50179.

U.S. Department of Health and Human Services. *The Health Consequences of Smoking: Chronic Obstructive Lung Disease. A Report of the Surgeon General.* Rock ville (MD): U.S. Department of Health and Human Services, Public Health Service, Office on Smoking and Health, 1984. DHHS Publication No. (PHS) 84 50205.

U.S. Department of Health and Human Services. *The Health Consequences of Involuntary Smoking. A Report of the Surgeon General.* Rockville (MD): U.S. Department of Health and Human Services, Public Health Service, Centers for Disease Control, Cen ter for Health Promotion and Education, Office on Smoking and Health, 1986. DHHS Publication No. (CDC) 87-8398.

U.S. Department of Health and Human Services. *Preventing Tobacco Use Among Young People. A Report of the Surgeon General.* Atlanta: U.S. Department of Health and Human Services, Public Health Ser vice, Centers for Disease Control and Prevention, National Center for Chronic Disease Prevention and Health Promotion, Office on Smoking and Health, 1994.

U.S. Department of Health and Human Services. *Tobacco Use Among U.S. Racial/Ethnic Minority Groups—African Americans, American Indians and Alaska Natives, Asian Americans and Pacific Islanders, and Hispanics. A Report of the Surgeon General.* Atlanta: U.S. Department of Health and Human Services, Centers for Disease Control and Preven tion, National Center for Chronic Disease Preven tion and Health Promotion, Office on Smoking and Health, 1998.

U.S. Department of Health and Human Services. *Women and Smoking. A Report of the Surgeon General.* Rockville (MD): U.S. Department of Health and Human Services, Public Health Service, Office of the Surgeon General, 2001.

U.S. Department of Health and Human Services. *The Health Consequences of Smoking: A Report of the Surgeon General.* Atlanta: U.S. Department of Health and Human Services, Centers for Disease Control and Prevention, National Center for Chronic Dis ease Prevention and Health Promotion, Office on Smoking and Health, 2004.

U.S. Department of Health and Human Services. *The Health Consequences of Involuntary Exposure to Tobacco Smoke: A Report of the Surgeon General.* Atlanta: U.S. Department of Health and Human Services, Cen ters for

Disease Control and Prevention, National Center for Chronic Disease Prevention and Health Promotion, Office on Smoking and Health, 2006.

U.S. Department of Health, Education, and Welfare. *Smoking and Health: Report of the Advisory Committee to the Surgeon General of the Public Health Service.* Washington: U.S. Department of Health, Education, and Welfare, Public Health Service, Center for Disease Control, 1964. PHS Publication No. 1103.

U.S. Department of Health, Education, and Welfare. *The Health Consequences of Smoking. A Report of the Surgeon General: 1972.* Washington: U.S. Department of Health, Education, and Welfare, Public Health Service, Health Services and Mental Health Administration, 1972. DHEW Publication No. (HSM) 72-7516.

U.S. Department of Health, Education, and Welfare. *The Health Consequences of Smoking. A Report of the Surgeon General, 1975.* Washington: U.S. Department of Health, Education, and Welfare, Public Health Service, Center for Disease Control, 1975. DHEW Publication No. (CDC) 77-8704.

U.S. Department of Health, Education, and Welfare. *Smoking and Health. A Report of the Surgeon General.* Washington: U.S. Department of Health, Education, and Welfare, Public Health Service, Office of the Assistant Secretary for Health, Office of Smoking and Health, 1979. DHEW Publication No. (PHS) 79-50066.

U.S. Environmental Protection Agency. *Respiratory Health Effects of Passive Smoking: Lung Cancer and Other Disorders.* Washington: U.S. Environmental Protection Agency, Office of Research and Development, Office of Air Radiation, 1992. Report No. EPA/600/6-90/0006F.

In: Children and Secondhand Smoke Exposure ISBN: 978-1-60692-587-4
Editor: J. R. Harrington © 2009 Nova Science Publishers, Inc.

Chapter 2

EXCERPTS FROM CHAPTER 4. PREVALENCE OF EXPOSURE TO SECONDHAND SMOKE

INTRODUCTION

The 1986 U.S. Surgeon General's report, *The Health Consequences of Involuntary Smoking*, outlined the need for valid and reliable methods to more accu rately determine and assess the health consequences of exposure to secondhand smoke (U.S. Department of Health and Human Services [USDHHS] 1986). The report concluded that reliable methods were neces sary to research the health effects and to characterize the public health impact of exposure to secondhand tobacco smoke in the home, at work, and in other environments. The report noted that without valid and reliable evidence, policymakers could not draft and implement effective policies to reduce and elimi nate exposures: "Validated questionnaires are needed for the assessment of recent and remote exposure to environmental tobacco smoke in the home, workplace, and other environments" (USDHHS 1986, p. 14).

Since the publication of that report, public health investigators have made significant advances in the development and application of reliable and valid research methods to assess exposure to secondhand smoke (Jaakkola and Samet 1999; Samet and Wang 2000). Several investigators have recently developed new methods to measure tobacco smoke concentrations in indoor environments and have discovered sensitive biologic markers of active and involuntary exposures (Jaakkola and Samet 1999; Samet and Wang 2000). These advances have generated a substantial amount of data on exposure of nonsmokers to secondhand smoke and have improved the capability of researchers to measure a recent exposure. However, many public health investigators agree that more accurate tools are still needed to measure temporally remote exposures, which, by necessity, are still assessed using questionnaires (Jaakkola and Samet 1999).

The main methods researchers rely on to evaluate secondhand smoke exposure are questionnaires, measurements of concentrations of the airborne components of secondhand smoke, and measurements of biomarkers (see Chapter 3, Assessment of Exposure to Secondhand Smoke in the full report). The discussion that follows on the prevalence of secondhand smoke exposure includes current metrics of exposure, changes in exposure over time, exposure of special populations such as children with asthma and persons in prisons, and international differences in exposure.

METHODS

To identify research publications on biomarkers of secondhand smoke, the authors of this chapter reviewed the published literature for studies on population exposures to and concentrations of secondhand smoke in different environments by conducting a Medline search with the following terms: tobacco smoke pollution, environmental tobacco smoke, and secondhand smoke. These terms were then paired with the term population or survey. The authors then reviewed abstracts of articles to specifically identify studies that used representative surveys of the U.S. population for inclusion in this report.

To specifically identify articles on concentrations of secondhand smoke, the authors used Boolean logic to search Medline and Web of Science, pairing the selected terms for secondhand smoke (second hand smoke, environmental tobacco smoke, passive smoking, and involuntary smoking) with terms indicative of a location that included home, work, work place, occupation and restaurants, bars, public places, sports, transportation, buses, trains, cars, airplanes, casinos, bingo, nightclubs, prisons, correctional institutions, nursing homes, and mental institutions. The authors searched for these terms with and without other selected terms such as exposure, concentration, and level of exposure. The authors also included data from a review of studies on the composition and measurement of secondhand smoke (Jenkins et al. 2000).

This chapter focuses on measured concentrations of airborne nicotine—nicotine is a specific tracer for secondhand smoke and has therefore been widely used in many studies. This discussion also focuses on biomarker levels of cotinine, the metabolite of nicotine. Thus, the abstracts of articles identified through the literature search were further reviewed for data that contained measured values of nicotine in the air of selected environments.

ESTIMATES OF EXPOSURE

National Trends in Biomarkers of Exposure

Beginning in 1988, researchers used serum coti nine measurements to assess exposures to secondhand smoke in the United States within the National Health and Nutrition Examination Survey (NHANES). The NHANES is conducted by the National Center for Health Statistics (NCHS), Centers for Disease Control and Prevention (CDC), and is designed to examine a nationally representative sample of the U.S. civilian (noninstitutionalized) population based upon a com plex, stratified, multistage probability cluster sam pling design (see http://www.cdc.gov/nchs/nhanes. htm). The protocols include a home interview fol lowed by a physical examination in a mobile examina tion center, where blood samples are drawn for serum cotinine analysis. NHANES III, conducted from 1988 to 1994, was the first national survey of secondhand smoke exposure of the entire U.S. population aged 4 through 74 years. There were two phases: Phase I from 1988 to 1991, and Phase II from 1991 to 1994. There were no further studies between 1995 and 1998. In 1999, NCHS resumed NHANES on a continuous basis and completed a new nationally representative sample every two years. This more recent NHANES (1999) also began to draw blood samples for serum cotinine analyses from participants aged three years and older.

Researchers have reported serum cotinine lev els in nonsmokers from the NHANES for four dis tinct intervals within the overall time period of 14 years, from 1988 through 2002: Phase I and Phase II of NHANES III, NHANES 1999–2000, and NHANES 2001–2002 (Pirkle et al. 1996, 2006). Researchers have reported additional data on serum cotinine lev els in nonsmokers from NHANES 1999–2002 in the National Report on Human Exposure to Environmen tal Chemicals (CDC 2001a, 2003, 2005). To maintain comparability among survey intervals, trend data are only reported for participants aged four or more years in each study interval (Pirkle et al. 2006). Factors that affect nicotine metabolism, such as age, race, and the level of exposure to secondhand smoke, also influence cotinine levels (Caraballo et al. 1998; Mannino et al. 2001). Because cotinine levels reflect exposures that occurred within two to three days, they represent pat terns of usual exposure (Jarvis et al. 1987; Benowitz 1996; Jaakkola and Jaakkola 1997).

Studies document NHANES serum cotinine levels in both children and adult nonsmokers (Pirkle et al. 1996, 2006; CDC 2001a, 2003, 2005). Nonsmoking adults were defined in these studies as persons whose serum cotinine concentrations were 10 nanograms per milliliter (ng/mL) or less, who reported no tobacco or nicotine use in the five days before the mobile examination center visit, and who were self-reported former smokers or lifetime nonsmokers. In NHANES III, the laboratory limit of detection was 0.050 ng/mL. However, the laboratory methods have continued to improve, and the detection limit was recently lowered to 0.015 ng/mL (CDC 2005; Pirkle et al. 2006). Additionally, researchers have categorized serum cotinine concentrations by age, race, and ethnicity. The racial and ethnic categories are non-Hispanic White, non-Hispanic Black, Mexican American, or "Other," and are self-reported. The category of "Other" was included in these reports in mean and percentile estimates for the total population but not in the geometric mean estimates because of small sample sizes (CDC 2005; Pirkle et al. 2006).

Figure 4.1 shows the overall proportion of all nonsmokers aged four or more years with serum cotinine levels of 0.050 ng/mL or greater for the four survey periods. Pirkle and colleagues (1996) reported detectable levels of serum cotinine among nearly all nonsmokers (87.9 percent) during Phase I (1988–1991) of NHANES III. Exposures among nonsmokers have declined significantly since that time (CDC 2005). The proportion of U.S. nonsmokers with cotinine concentrations of 0.050 ng/mL or greater fell to 43 percent in NHANES 2001–2002 (Pirkle et al. 2006).

Pirkle and colleagues (2006) provided additional data on the levels and distribution of serum cotinine concentrations in U.S. nonsmokers during 1988–2002. Trends in the adjusted geometric mean cotinine concentrations (adjusted for age, race, and gender) are in table 4.1. Since Phase I of NHANES III, secondhand smoke exposures measured by serum cotinine concentrations in U.S. nonsmokers aged four or more years have declined by about 75 percent (from 0.247 ng/mL to 0.061 ng/mL). While declines among children aged 4 through 11 years and young persons aged 12 through 19 years also have been notable, the declines have been smaller than those among adults aged 20 through 74 years. Trends among racial and ethnic categories were also stratified by age: 4 through 11 years, 12 through 19 years, and 20 through 74 years. Pirkle and colleagues (2006) noted that serum cotinine levels in NHANES differed by race and ethnicity. Overall, in the order of the adjusted mean cotinine concentrations during each of the four time periods, concentrations among Mexican Americans were less than those of non-Hispanic Whites, which were less than those of non-Hispanic Blacks; the non-

Hispanic Black mean cotinine concentrations were significantly higher during each of the four time periods (Pirkle et al. 2006).

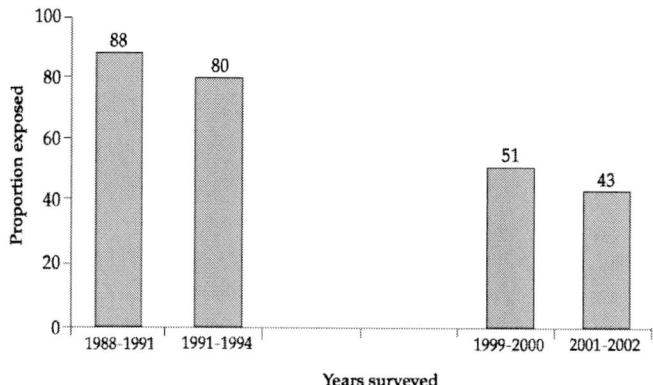

Source: Adapted from Pirkle et al. 2006. [1] Serum contine ≥0.05 nanograms per milliliter. [2] Aged ≥4 years. [3] NHANES=national Health and Nutrition Examination Survey.

Figure 4.1. Trends in exposure1 of nonsmokers2 to secondhand smoke in the U.S. population, NHANES3 1988-2002.

Current patterns of secondhand smoke exposure are reflected in the NHANES 1999–2002 serum cotinine concentrations (table 4.2). As noted in fgure 4.1, the proportion of U.S. nonsmokers with serum cotinine levels of 0.050 ng/mL or greater has declined since NHANES III to less than 45 percent. However, the proportion of children and nonsmoking adults with serum cotinine levels of 0.050 ng/mL or greater in NHANES 1999–2002 differs significantly by age, from 59.6 percent among children aged 3 through 11 years to 35.7 percent among nonsmoking adults aged 60 through 74 years. Additionally, the median cotinine concentration in the serum is significantly higher in children aged 3 through 11 years (0.09 ng/mL) than in older adults (0.035 ng/mL) (CDC 2005). Children aged 3 through 11 years and youth aged 12 through 19 years are also significantly more likely than adults to live in a household with at least one smoker. Estimates of the number of secondhand smoke exposures nationwide in 2000 can be extrapolated from national estimates of the proportion of children and nonsmoking adults with measured serum cotinine concentrations of 0.05 ng/mL or greater. Overall, based upon serum cotinine measures, approximately 22 million children aged 3 through 11 years, 18 million nonsmoking youth aged 12 through 19 years, and 86 million nonsmoking adults aged 20 or more years in the United States were exposed to secondhand smoke in 2000 (table 4.2).

Table 4.1. Trends in serum cotinine levels (nanograms per milliliter) of nonsmokers* stratified by age, gender, race, and ethnicity, United States, 1988–2002

Population		NHANES III, Phase I 1988–1991	NHANES III, Phase II 1991–1994	NHANES 1999–2000	NHANES 2001–2002	% decline from 1988–1991 to 2001–2002
Overall	Geometric mean†	0.247	0.182	0.106	0.061	75.3
	95% CI‡	0.219–0.277	0.165–0.202	0.094–0.119	0.049–0.076	
Aged ~4 years						
Aged 4–11 years						
Male	Geometric mean	0.283	0.234	0.166	0.098	65.4
	95% CI	0.223–0.360	0.188–0.291	0.105–0.262	0.064–0.151	
Female	Geometric mean	0.328	0.285	0.172	0.115	64.9
	95% CI	0.240–0.449	0.235–0.345	0.113–0.262	0.075–0.177	
Race and ethnicity						
Non-Hispanic White	Geometric mean	0.295	0.255	0.171	0.100	
	95% CI	0.226–0.385	0.214–0.303	0.100–0.293	0.061–0.165	
Non-Hispanic Black	Geometric mean	0.534	0.460	0.284	0.261	
	95% CI	0.387–0.738	0.393–0.538	0.249–0.324	0.188–0.361	
Mexican American	Geometric mean	0.192	0.125	0.080	0.060	
	95% CI	0.148–0.250	0.107–0.145	0.066–0.097	0.042–0.086	
Aged 12–19 years						

Population		NHANES III, Phase I 1988–1991	NHANES III, Phase II 1991–1994	NHANES 1999–2000	NHANES 2001–2002	% decline from 1988–1991 to 2001–2002
Male	Geometric mean	0.346	0.239	0.189	0.090	74.0
	95% CI	0.255–0.470	0.190–0.300	0.138–0.258	0.061–0.132	
Female	Geometric mean	0.280	0.228	0.156	0.078	72.1
	95% CI	0.223–0.353	0.175–0.298	0.124–0.197	0.048–0.126	
Race and ethnicity						
Non-Hispanic White	Geometric mean	0.301	0.219	0.170	0.074	
	95% CI	0.228–0.396	0.174–0.276	0.139–0.210	0.044–0.123	
Non-Hispanic Black	Geometric mean	0.515	0.460	0.263	0.227	
	95% CI	0.392–0.677	0.374–0.567	0.229–0.303	0.191–0.270	
Mexican American	Geometric mean	0.179	0.143	0.095	0.063	
	95% CI	0.139–0.229	0.126–0.162	0.082–0.110	0.045–0.089	
Aged ~20 years						
Male	Geometric mean	0.293	0.199	0.106	0.067	77.1
	95% CI	0.259–0.332	0.178–0.222	0.092–0.122	0.054–0.082	
Female	Geometric mean	0.188	0.138	0.078	0.042	77.7
	95% CI	0.165–0.215	0.120–0.159	0.072–0.085	0.035–0.050	
Race and ethnicity						
Non-Hispanic White	Geometric mean	0.215	0.151	0.085	0.044	

Table 4.1. (Continued).

Population		NHANES III, Phase I 1988–1991	NHANES III, Phase II 1991–1994	NHANES 1999–2000	NHANES 2001–2002	% decline from 1988–1991 to 2001–2002
	95% CI	0.189–0.244	0.133–0.172	0.077–0.095	0.036–0.055	
Non-Hispanic Black	Geometric mean	0.401	0.299	0.135	0.129	
	95% CI	0.325–0.494	0.271–0.330	0.116–0.157	0.101–0.163	
Mexican American	Geometric mean	0.204	0.138	0.078	0.058	
	95% CI	0.165–0.251	0.117–0.162	0.066–0.093	0.040–0.083	

*From four National Health and Nutrition Examination Survey (NHANES) study intervals.

† Individuals with serum cotinine levels below the laboratory limit of detection (LOD) were assigned a value of LOD/square root of 2.

‡ CI = Confidence interval.

Source: Adapted from Pirkle et al. 2006.

Although the number of children and nonsmoking adults currently exposed to secondhand smoke in the United States remains very large, there have been significant declines in the proportion and mean concentrations of these exposures since 1988. In order to characterize these trends in exposure, data on the principal environments where children and nonsmoking adults are typically exposed to secondhand smoke are reviewed in the discussion that follows.

Environmental Sites of Exposure

The principal places where studies have measured exposures to secondhand smoke represent key microenvironments: homes, worksites, and public places such as restaurants, malls, and bars. The contributions of these different locations to total personal exposures vary across different groups. For example, the dominant site of exposure for children is the home, whereas worksites are typically important exposure locations for nonsmoking adults who may not be exposed at home.

People spend most of their time at home, which is potentially the most important location of secondhand smoke exposure for people who live with regular smokers (Klepeis 1999). Because the workplace is second only to the home as the location where adults spend most of their time, smoking in the workplace has been a major contributor to total secondhand smoke exposure. The National Human Activity Pattern Survey (NHAPS), conducted from 1992 to 1994, interviewed 9,386 randomly chosen U.S. residents about their activities and exposures to secondhand smoke (Klepeis 1999; Klepeis et al. 2001). For those persons reporting secondhand smoke exposure of at least one minute, the average daily duration of the exposure and the percentage of respondents who reported an exposure in each indoor locale were as follows:

- 305 minutes in the home (58 percent);
- 363 minutes in the office or factory (10 percent);
- 249 minutes in schools or public buildings (6 percent);
- 143 minutes in bars or restaurants (23 percent);
- 198 minutes in malls or stores (7 percent);
- 79 minutes in vehicles (33 percent); and
- 255 minutes in other indoor locations (6 percent) (Klepeis 1999).

Table 4.2. Serum cotinine levels among nonsmokers aged 3 years and older, NHANES* 1999–2002

Age group	Median cotinine level (SE[†]) (95% CI[‡])	% with levels ≥ 0.05 ng/mL[§] (SE) (95% CI)	% with at least 1 smoker in the home (SE) (95% CI)	Total population (2000)	Estimated number of persons (in millions) with serum cotinine levels ≥ 0.05 ng/mL
≥ 3 years	<LOD (<LOD–0.52)	47.0 (1.9) (43.0–50.9)	11.1 (0.45) (10.2–12.0)	270,005,230	126.9
3–19 years	0.08 (0.01) (0.06–0.11)	57.7 (2.8) (52.0–63.3)	22.6 (1.4) (19.9–25.6)	69,056,589	39.8
3–11 years	0.09 (0.02) (0.06–0.12)	59.6 (2.9) (53.5–65.4)	24.9 (1.8) (21.5–28.7)	36,697,776	21.9
12–19 years	0.07 (0.01) (0.05–0.10)	55.6 (3.1) (49.1–61.9)	19.9 (1.3) (17.4–22.7)	32,358,813	18.0
≥ 20 years	<LOD (<LOD–<LOD)	42.8 (1.9) (39.0–46.6)	6.56 (0.32) (5.93–7.25)	200,948,641	86.0
20–39 years	<LOD (<LOD–0.066)	49.2 (2.9) (43.3–55.2)	6.85 (0.77) (5.43–8.61)	81,562,389	40.1
40–59 years	<LOD (<LOD–<LOD)	41.6 (2.2) (37.1–46.2)	7.3 (0.86) (5.73–9.26)	73,589,052	30.6
≥ 60 years	<LOD (<LOD–<LOD)	35.7 (1.7) (32.3–39.4)	5.12 (0.52) (4.15–6.3)	45,797,200	16.3

*NHANES = National Health and Nutrition Examination Survey.
[†]SE = Standard error.
[‡]CI = Confidence interval.
[§]ng/mL = Nanograms per milliliter.
LOD = Limit of detection (0.05 ng/mL).
Sources: U.S. Bureau of the Census 2005; Centers for Disease Control and Prevention, National Center for Health Statistics, unpublished data.

Even for adults who live in homes where smoking routinely occurs, the workplace can add significantly to this exposure. Among NHANES III participants who lived in smoke-free homes, a work place that permitted smoking was typically the major contributor to their total secondhand smoke exposure (Pirkle et al. 1996).

Studies have shown that restaurants can be important sites of exposures to children as well as adults (Maskarinec et al. 2000; McMillen et al. 2003; Skeer and Siegel 2003; Siegel et al. 2004), and other public places may also contribute substantially to exposures of selected segments of the population. Finally, persons who cannot move about freely, such as those who live in nursing homes, mental institu tions, or correctional facilities, may find such expo sures unavoidable.

Exposure in the Home

Secondhand smoke exposure at home can be substantial for both children and adults (Jenkins et al. 1996a; Pirkle et al. 1996; Klepeis 1999; Klepeis et al. 2001). This section considers children exposed to sec ondhand smoke at home separately from adults who are exposed at home because the patterns are different for the two groups (Mannino et al. 1996, 1997). The definition of "children" varies across the studies cited in this report. There are also separate data for special populations, including children with asthma, preg nant women, and persons living in the inner city.

Representative Surveys of Children

Researchers have conducted a number of local (Greenberg et al. 1989), state (King et al. 1998), and national (Mannino et al. 1996) surveys of childhood exposure to secondhand smoke. One of the best data sources available on children's secondhand smoke exposure in the home is the National Health Inter view Survey (NHIS). This information can be derived from NHIS data by correlating data on smoking in the home with data on households with children. NHIS data shows that the proportion of children aged 6 years and younger who are regularly exposed to sec ondhand smoke in their homes fell from 27 percent in 1994 to 20 percent in 1998. Most surveys were pri marily based on the indirect indicator of one or more smoking adults in a home; estimates of the percent ages exposed in the home ranged from 54 to 75 per cent of the children (Lebowitz and Burrows

1976; Schilling et al. 1977; Ferris et al. 1985). A 1988 survey using an indirect indicator estimated that 48.9 percent of the children studied had experienced postnatal exposures to secondhand smoke (Overpeck and Moss 1991). Exposure prevalence was higher for children in poverty (63.6 percent) or for those whose mothers had less than 12 years of education (66.7 percent). An analysis of National Health Interview Survey (NHIS) data for 1994 showed that 35 percent of U.S. children lived in homes where they had contact with a smoker at least one day per week (Schuster et al. 2002).

Use of the indirect approach assumes that the presence of a smoking adult in the household results in exposure of children to secondhand smoke. Over time, as more people recognized the health effects from exposure in the home and implemented in-home smoking policies, the presence of smoking adults in the home has become a less valid indicator of expo sure. In a 1991 survey of U.S. adults, 11.8 percent of current smokers reported that because no smoking had occurred in their homes in the two weeks before the survey, their children had not been exposed to secondhand smoke in the home (Mannino et al. 1996). Using data from the California Tobacco Survey, Gilpin and colleagues (2001) found that the proportion of households prohibiting smoking increased from 50.9 percent in 1993 to 72.8 percent in 1999 (Gilpin et al. 2001). The increase was greater in homes with smokers, from 20.1 percent in 1993 to 47.2 percent in 1999 (Pierce et al. 1998; Gilpin et al. 2001). The survey did not capture data from nonfamily members who may have smoked in the home, nor would it have addressed the contamination of one dwelling from smokers in another within a multiresidence building.

Other analyses have used questionnaires that ask specifically about the number of cigarettes smoked in the home to determine whether children were exposed to secondhand smoke. A 1991 nation ally representative survey estimated that 31.2 percent of U.S. children were exposed daily to secondhand smoke in their homes, with an additional 5.8 percent exposed at home at least one day in the previous two weeks (Mannino et al. 1996). This exposure varied significantly by socioeconomic status (SES) (46.5 per cent for a lower SES versus 22.5 percent for a higher SES) and by region of the country, with the lowest exposure (24.3 percent) in the western part of the United States (Mannino et al. 1996). In Phase I of the NHANES III (collected from 1988 to 1991), 43 percent of children aged 2 months through 11 years lived in a home with at least one smoker (Pirkle et al. 1996). In NHANES 1999–2002, the proportion of children aged 3 through 11 years living with one or more smokers in the household was 24.9 percent (table 4.2). However, 59.6 percent of children aged 3 through 11 years had a serum cotinine concentration of 0.05 ng/mL or higher. State and local surveys have documented higher lev els of reported exposure. In a 1985 study from New Mexico, 60 to 70 percent of the children had been exposed to secondhand smoke (Coultas et al. 1987). In a 1986 study of North Carolina infants, 56 percent had been exposed (Margolis et al. 1997). On the basis of self-reported data on smoking among household resi dents, CDC estimated in 1996 that 21.9 percent of U.S. children had been exposed to secondhand smoke in their homes (CDC 1997). The prevalence of exposure varied by state, from a low of 11.7 percent in Utah to a high of 34.2 percent in Kentucky. However, the data on serum cotinine concentrations suggest that these estimates are low.

As noted above, since 1988 the NHANES has provided nationally representative measurements of serum cotinine levels in both children and adults (Pirkle et al. 1996, 2006; CDC 2001a, 2003, 2005). Table 4.1 shows overall U.S. trends in exposure measured by serum cotinine concentrations. Although exposures have declined among both children and adults since Phase I of NHANES III (1988–1991), the percentage of the decline was smaller among children aged 4 through 11 years. In the NHANES 2001–2002, mean cotinine levels were highest among children aged 4 through 11 years (non-Hispanic Black children in particular) (Pirkle et al. 2006). Measured cotinine concentrations were more than twice as high among children aged 4 through 11 years than among nonsmoking adults aged 20 or more years, and the levels of non-Hispanic Black children were two to three times higher than those of non-Hispanic White and Mexican American children. While metabolic factors can also influence cotinine levels (Caraballo et al. 1998; Mannino et al. 2001), the racial and ethnic differences in serum cotinine con centrations overall, and particularly among children, presumably reflect greater exposures to secondhand smoke among non-Hispanic Black populations (Pirkle et al. 2006).

Table 4.2 compares current estimates of national exposure by age. In Phases I and II of NHANES III (1988–1994), 84.7 percent of children aged 4 through 11 years had a serum cotinine concentration of 0.05 ng/mL or greater; 99.1 percent of children with a reported exposure in the home and 75.6 percent of children without any reported exposure had measur able cotinine levels (Mannino et al. 2001). The stron gest predictor of cotinine levels in children was the number of cigarettes smoked daily in the home, but other factors were also significant predictors, includ ing race, ethnicity, age of the child, size of the home, and region of the country (Mannino et al. 2001). In the most recent estimates of exposure (table 4.2), 59.6 per cent of children aged 3 through 11 years had a serum cotinine concentration of 0.05 ng/mL or greater, and 24.9 percent reported living with at least one smoker in the household. Based upon this estimate of the pro portion of children aged 3 through 11 years living with a smoker in the household, an estimated nine million children or more in this age range may be exposed to secondhand smoke. However, serum cotinine mea surements indicate an even greater exposed popula tion of almost 22 million children aged 3 through 11 years in the year 2000.

Trends in exposure of children to secondhand smoke indicate that levels of exposure have declined significantly since Phase I of NHANES III (Pirkle et al. 2006). The multiple factors related to this decline are still being studied. Several researchers have suggested that a major component of this decline is related to the decrease in parental smoking (Shopland et al. 1996) and to the increase in household smoking restrictions (Gilpin et al. 2001). Data from the 1992 and 2000 NHIS (Soliman et al. 2004) indicate that self-reported expo sure of nonsmokers to secondhand smoke in homes with children declined significantly in the 1990s from 36 percent in 1992 to 25 percent in 2000. Because researchers have identified parental smoking in the home as a major source for exposure among younger children (Mannino et al. 2001), this decline in reported home exposures to secondhand smoke suggests that voluntary changes in home policies and smoking practices of adults in homes where children reside are a major contributing factor to the observed declines in serum cotinine concentrations among children since Phase I of NHANES III.

Protecting children from secondhand smoke exposure in homes has been the focus of the U.S. Envi ronmental Protection Agency's parental outreach and educational programs to promote smoke-free home rules for the last decade. The potential for exposing children to secondhand smoke has dropped even further as more local and state governments restrict smoking in public areas (CDC 1999). Jarvis and col leagues (2000) documented similar findings in data from Great Britain. From 1988 to 1996, the proportion of homes without smokers increased from 48 to 55 percent. During this same period, the geometric mean salivary cotinine levels decreased from 0.47 to 0.28 ng/mL among children with nonsmoking parents, and from 3.08 to 2.25 ng/mL among children with two smoking parents (Jarvis et al. 2000).

Additional studies that document exposure of children in the United States to secondhand smoke in the home include three studies that reported the pres ence of some form of smoking ban at home in many households (Norman et al. 1999; Kegler and Malcoe 2002; McMillen et al. 2003). Norman and colleagues (1999) surveyed a representative sample of 6,985 Cali fornia adults. Kegler and Malcoe (2002) studied 380 rural, low-income Native American and White par ents from northeastern Oklahoma. McMillan and col leagues (2003) conducted a telephone survey of more than 4,500 eligible adults across the United States. Two other studies also focused on prevalence and patterns of childhood household secondhand smoke exposure in the United States: CDC (2001b) reported on the Behavioral Risk Factor Surveillance System (BRFSS) telephone interviews that took place in 20 states, and Schuster and colleagues (2002) reported on personal interviews with 45,335 respondents from around the country in the 1994 NHIS.

Susceptible Populations

Some populations may be particularly susceptible to secondhand smoke exposure. Examples include persons with asthma or other chronic respiratory diseases, and fetuses exposed to tobacco smoke components in utero either by maternal smoking or maternal exposure to secondhand smoke. In one 1994 community-based study in Seattle, 31 percent of children with asthma reported household exposures to secondhand smoke, but only 17 percent of children without asthma reported an exposure (Maier et al. 1997).

Studies have tracked smoking by pregnant women using several different data collection systems including natality surveys, NHIS, BRFSS, National Survey of Family Growth, and since 1989, birth certificates in nearly all states and the District of Columbia (CDC 2001a). The estimates from these different sources generally agree that the proportion of women who report smoking during pregnancy has decreased in recent years, from between 30 and 40 percent in the early 1980s to between 10 and 15 percent in the late 1990s. By 2003, only an estimated 10.7 percent of mothers of a live-born infant reported smoking during pregnancy. However, the prevalence of reported smoking was not uniform across all population groups or education levels. For example, a CDC report (CDC 2005) documented that 18 percent of American Indian or Alaska Native women reported smoking during pregnancy, but only 3 percent of Hispanic women reported smoking during pregnancy. And women with 9 to 11 years of education were far more likely to report smoking (25.5 percent) compared with women with 16 or more years of education (1.6 percent) (CDC 2005). Ebrahim and colleagues (2000) showed that the declining trend in smoking during pregnancy in recent years is primarily attributable to a decrease in smoking prevalence among women of childbearing age, rather than to an increase in smoking cessation during pregnancy. Of the women who reported smoking during pregnancy, most (68.6 percent) said that they had smoked 10 or fewer cigarettes daily.

Researchers have also found that pregnant women may conceal their smoking from clinicians (Windsor et al. 1993; Ford et al. 1997). Thus, smoking during pregnancy may be underestimated. Estimates of the prevalence of smoking during pregnancy are also sensitive to how smoking was defined in a study, which may range from any smoking at any time during pregnancy to smoking during the final three months of pregnancy.

Complicating the interpretation of findings on health effects of secondhand smoke exposure in very young children is evidence that a large proportion of children are exposed both prenatally and postnatally. Overpeck and Moss (1991) used CDC data to show that 96 percent of children with prenatal exposures also had postnatal exposures. The investigators found that 29 percent of the children had been exposed prenatally to maternal smoking and that an additional 21 percent had been exposed to secondhand smoke postnatally. A second source of involuntary smoking for a developing fetus is the exposure of a pregnant woman to secondhand smoke. The factors that predicted prenatal maternal exposure to secondhand smoke were similar to those associated with second hand smoke exposure in general, such as low SES, low levels of education, and living in a small home (Overpeck and Moss 1991).

Although national surveys have not specifically asked about secondhand smoke exposure during pregnancy, they have provided estimates of exposure among women of childbearing age. In NHANES III, 18 percent of nonsmoking females aged 17 years and older reported exposures to secondhand smoke. However, the percentages of reported exposures were higher among women of childbearing age: 31 percent for 17- through 19-year-olds, 30 percent for 20- through 29-year-olds, and 26 percent for 30- through 39-year olds (Pirkle et al. 1996). Of the nontobacco users surveyed in 1988–1991, 88 percent had detectable levels of serum cotinine (>0.050 ng/mL), a finding that suggests an unreported or unknown exposure. These findings are consistent with results from a 1985 study of 1,231 nonsmoking pregnant women in Maine, which found that 70 percent of the participants had cotinine levels above 0.5 ng/mL (Haddow et al. 1987).

Measurements of Airborne Tracers in Homes

Numerous studies have measured secondhand smoke concentrations in homes (Leaderer and Hammond 1991; Hammond et al. 1993; Marbury et al. 1993; Manning et al. 1994; O'Connor et al. 1995; Jenkins et al. 1996a,b; Phillips et al. 1996, 1997a,b, 1998a–h, 1999a,b). Concentrations of secondhand smoke components are higher at the time that the cigarettes are smoked compared with a few hours later. Measurements taken only during periods of smoking document higher concentrations than samples measured during both smoking and nonsmoking periods. For example, Muramatsu and colleagues (1984) measured both nicotine and particulate matter sequentially for 10 hours in an office. They found that the 30-minute nicotine samples ranged from 2 to 26 micrograms per cubic meter (jig/m^3) during the workday; most values ranged between 5 and 15 jig/m^3. The 10-hour averaged concentration was 10 jig/m^3, which was based on a shorter time period than that used by other studies to obtain stable estimates. Most studies have measured concentrations averaged over longer periods of time, which include periods with and without smoking.

Studies have demonstrated a high correlation (Spearman rho correlation coefficient = 0.74, p <0.001) between nicotine concentrations measured in the family activity rooms and in the kitchens (Emmons et al. 2001), as well as between concentrations in the activity rooms and in the bedrooms (Spearman correlation coefficient = 0.91; 0.90 for homes of smokers only) (Marbury et al. 1993).

The results of several studies that measured nicotine concentrations in the homes of smokers in the United States are presented in the full report (see figure 4.2 and table 4.3). Median nicotine concentrations were generally between 1 and 3 jig/m^3 (averaged over 14 hours to several weeks), with nicotine concentrations ranging from <0.1 to 8 jig/m^3 across the span from minimum to the 95th percentile. An exception was a study of 291 low-income homes in New England that found 4 homes with concentrations above 18 jig/m^3 (Emmons et al. 2001). Homes where smoking was restricted to the basement or the outdoors had lower mean nicotine concentrations of 0.3 jig/m^3 (Marbury et al. 1993).

Personal sampling of secondhand smoke exposure has yielded similar results with measured home exposure. In a study of exposure away from work (predominantly at home, lasting 16 hours), 306 nonsmokers who reported secondhand smoke exposure had a mean nicotine exposure of 2.7 jig/m^3 (median 1.2 jig/m^3), with a 95th percentile value of 7.9 in 1993 and 1994 (Jenkins et al. 1996a). Personal sampling of 100 people in Massachusetts during 1987 and 1988 found the median of a weekly average of nicotine concentrations to be 1.0 jig/m^3 for nonsmokers married to nonsmokers and 3.5 jig/m^3 for those married to smokers; the respective maximum values were 9.5 and 14 jig/m^3. These values included all exposures throughout the week in homes, workplaces, and public places (Coghlin et al. 1989, 1991). To evaluate secondhand smoke exposure among pregnant women, participants in two studies wore passive samplers (small personal monitors that measure secondhand smoke exposure) for one week. Although the two studies had similar designs, the investigators reported quite different results. Among 36 low-income pregnant women in Massachusetts, 80 percent were exposed to nicotine at 0.5 jig/m^3 or greater, and 25 percent were exposed at a concentration above 2.0 jig/m^3 (Hammond et al. 1993). The measured exposure was lower for 131 pregnant upper-middle-class women in Connecticut who reported secondhand smoke exposure, with a median of 0.1 jig/m^3 and a 90th percentile of 0.6 jig/m^3 (O'Connor et al. 1995).

International studies of secondhand smoke expo sure sponsored by the tobacco industry (Jenkins et al. 1996a; Phillips et al. 1996, 1997a,b, 1998a–h, 1999a,b) followed a similar protocol where participants wore a sampling device for 16 to 24 hours. Figure 4.3 in the full report illustrates the median nicotine concentra tions observed "away from work" (predominantly at home) in the United States compared with homes in Australia and in several European and Asian loca tions. U.S. homes had the second highest reported values after Beijing, which reported a median of 1.3 jig/m^3. Hong Kong homes reported 0.3 jig/m^3, which was consistent with a study of 300 Chinese homes in 18 provinces that reported a 0.1 jig/m^3 weekly aver age concentration of nicotine in the homes of smokers (Hammond 1999).

Exposure in Public Places

Exposures to secondhand smoke in public places have been particular public health concerns for more than two decades. Although these sites are workplaces for some, they may now be the only source of second hand smoke exposure for most of the U.S. population with no home or work exposures. Studies using bio markers confirm that secondhand smoke exposure in public places continues to affect nonsmokers. Using NHANES III data, several investigators have shown that persons with no home or workplace exposures still had detectable levels of cotinine in their serum (Pirkle et al. 1996; Mannino et al. 2001). This finding suggests that many people are exposed to secondhand smoke in other locations.

Restaurants, Cafeterias, and Bars

Restaurants, cafeterias, and bars are worksites as well as public places where smoking is frequently unrestricted or restricted in a manner that does not effectively decrease exposure. Servers and bartenders working in environments where smoking is permitted may be exposed to high levels of secondhand smoke (Jarvis et al. 1992; Jenkins and Counts 1999). In a sur vey of 1,224 residents from Olmsted County, Minne sota, 57 percent of the respondents reported exposures to secondhand smoke: 44 percent reported exposures in restaurants, 21 percent reported exposures at work, and 19 percent reported exposures in bars (Kottke et al. 2001). A quarter of the respondents in the NHAPS study reported exposures in restaurants or bars on the previous day for an average of two and one-half hours (Klepeis 1999; Klepeis et al. 2001). Restaurants may be the principal point of secondhand smoke exposure for children from nonsmoking homes, and an exposure of even a short duration may be relevant to acute effects, such as inducing or exacerbating an asthma attack.

In eating establishments, a wide variability in factors determines the concentration of secondhand smoke, including the size of the room, ventilation rate, number of smokers, and smoking rate. Further more, these concentrations vary throughout the day and evening. Concentrations measured for one to two hours during lunch or dinner are likely to be much higher than the average concentrations measured during a full day or week. The nicotine concentrations measured in restaurants have ranged from less than detectable to values of 70 jig/m^3.

Tobacco smoke has long been considered a nuisance that interferes with the enjoyment of food. One approach to reducing exposures of nonsmokers has been to establish smoking and nonsmoking sec tions in restaurants. Nonsmoking sections generally do have lower concentrations of secondhand smoke (Lambert et al. 1993; Hammond 1999), but they nei ther eliminate secondhand smoke nor reduce second hand smoke concentrations to insignificant levels. The concentrations of nicotine in nonsmoking sections of restaurants persist at high levels. For example, a study of seven restaurants in Albuquerque, New Mexico, found that half of them had concentrations above 1 jig/m^3 in the nonsmoking sections (Lambert et al. 1993). Similar results were noted in more than half of 71 restaurants surveyed in Indiana where nicotine concentrations were above 2 jig/m^3 in the nonsmok ing sections (Hammond and Perrino 2002). In a study of waiters exposed to secondhand smoke, the average nicotine concentration was as high as 5.8 jig/m^3, with the upper end of the range at 68 jig/m^3 (Maskarinec et al. 2000).

Hammond (1999) reported that nicotine concen trations in cafeterias were somewhat higher than in restaurants; average values were between 6 and 14 jig/m^3. Out of the 37 samples from company cafeterias in Massachusetts that allowed or restricted workplace smoking, two-thirds had nicotine concentrations that were above 5 jig/m^3. Secondhand smoke concentra tions measured during lunchtime at a medical center cafeteria revealed large gradients between the smok ing and nonsmoking sections. The concentrations were generally 25 to 40 jig/m^3 in the smoking section, 2 to 5 jig/m^3 in a nonsmoking section that was within 25 feet of the smoking section, and less than 0.5 jig/ m3 in a nonsmoking section that was 30 feet from the smoking section (although on one day, the average in that section was 1.8 jig/m^3).

Evidence Synthesis

Since 1986, investigators have reported a sub stantial amount of new evidence on exposure to secondhand smoke. The more recent data provide insights into typical patterns of exposure, exposure in key microenvironments, and the consequences of var ious policies intended to reduce exposure. As noted in table 4.1, exposures of nonsmokers to secondhand smoke have declined significantly between 1988 and 2002. These declines have been observed in both chil dren and nonsmoking adults, in both men and women, and in all racial and ethnic categories. However, sig nificant levels of exposure persist for the U.S. popula tion in general and for susceptible populations. Table 4.2 notes estimates for 2000; approximately 127 mil lion children and nonsmoking adults were exposed to secondhand smoke. This estimated total includes almost 22 million children aged 3 through 11 years, and 18 million nonsmoking youth aged 12 through 19 years.

The findings consistently show the importance of two microenvironments as places for second hand smoke exposure: the home and the workplace. Although microenvironments such as bars and res taurants may also be important for patrons, the home and the workplace are particularly significant because of the amount of time spent in these two locations. For the workplace, restrictions and smoking bans lead to much lower concentrations of secondhand smoke than in locations where smoking is allowed.

National surveys indicate that progress in reducing secondhand smoke exposure has been vari able across the country. Certain states, such as Cali fornia, Maryland, and Utah, have made significant advances in protecting nonsmokers, but others, such as Kentucky and Nevada, have not (Gilpin et al. 2001; Shopland et al. 2001). Even in locales with smoking restrictions in place, significant pockets of exposure remain, most notably in homes, some worksites such as restaurants and bars, and in automobiles. Expo sures in some of these locations can be remedied by changing public policy. Exposures in other locations, particularly homes and automobiles, can perhaps only be addressed through education that alters life style behaviors.

It is likely that geographic differences in second hand smoke exposure are related to trends in tobacco use and policies that determine where tobacco use is permitted (Giovino et al. 1995; Gilpin et al. 2001). Wide regional differences exist within the United States in secondhand smoke exposure and cotinine levels. In the NHANES III data, children with and without reported exposures had lower cotinine levels if they lived in the western part of the United States (Mannino et al. 2001)—a finding that may reflect lower community exposures to secondhand smoke.

Where smoking is allowed, especially at worksites and in public places, concentrations are highly vari able, so concentrations in individual locations may be significantly higher than average. Concentrations of secondhand smoke are also typically higher in the workplace and in restaurants than in the home. Poli cies that restrict smoking to particular areas reduce but do not eliminate secondhand smoke exposure. Smoke-free polices reduce secondhand smoke con centrations far more effectively.

CONCLUSIONS

The following conclusions are supported by text in the full report that may not be included in this excerpt. The full report can be accessed at http://www.surgeongeneral.gov/library/second handsmoke/report/.

1. The evidence is sufficient to infer that large numbers of nonsmokers are still exposed to secondhand smoke.
2. Exposure of nonsmokers to secondhand smoke has declined in the United States since the 1986 Surgeon General's report, *The Health Consequences of Involuntary Smoking.*
3. The evidence indicates that the extent of secondhand smoke exposure varies across the country.
4. Homes and workplaces are the predominant locations for exposure to secondhand smoke.
5. Exposure to secondhand smoke tends to be greater for persons with lower incomes.
6. Exposure to secondhand smoke continues in restaurants, bars, casinos, gaming halls, and vehicles.

OVERALL IMPLICATIONS

Exposure to secondhand smoke remains a seri ous public health problem in the United States, with exposure of almost 60 percent of children aged 3 through 11 years and more than 40 percent of non smoking adults. Since the publication of the 1986 Sur geon General's report, measured levels of exposure in the United States have declined significantly. How ever, the proportional decrease has been larger among adults than among children, and the most recent data suggest that children aged 3 through 11 years have serum cotinine concentrations that are more than twice as high as those among nonsmoking adults. Data sug gest that the home remains the most important target for reducing exposures to secondhand smoke, partic ularly for children but also for middle-aged and older adults. Although progress has been made to protect nonsmoking workers, continuing efforts are needed to protect these workers, and particularly younger workers, in all occupational categories.

Research questions remain regarding exposure to secondhand smoke. As noted in the 1986 report, no indicator has been developed that can objectively estimate long-term exposure or early-life expo sure. Secondhand smoke exposure from "shared air spaces" within a building is also of concern, as a sig nificant proportion of the population lives in apart ment buildings or condominiums where smoking in another part of the building might increase tobacco smoke exposure for households of nonsmokers.

REFERENCES

Benowitz NL. Cotinine as a biomarker of environmen tal tobacco smoke exposure. *Epidemiologic Reviews.* 1996;18(2):188–204.

Caraballo RS, Giovino GA, Pechacek TF, Mowery PD, Richter PA, Strauss WJ, Sharp DJ, Eriksen MP, Pirkle JL, Maurer KR. Racial and ethnic differences in serum cotinine levels of cigarette smokers: Third National Health and Nutrition Examination Sur vey, 1988–1991. *Journal of the American Medical Association.* 1998;280(2):135–9.

Centers for Disease Control and Prevention. State- specific prevalence of cigarette smoking among adults, and children's and adolescents' expo sure to environmental tobacco smoke—United States, 1996. *Morbidity and Mortality Weekly Report.* 1997;46(44):1038–43.

Centers for Disease Control and Prevention. State laws on tobacco control—United States, 1998. *Morbidity and Mortality Weekly Report.* 1999;48(3):21–40.

Centers for Disease Control and Prevention. *National Report on Human Exposure to Environmental Chemicals.* Atlanta: U.S. Department of Health and Human Services, Centers for Disease Control and Prevention, 2001a.

Centers for Disease Control and Prevention. State- specific prevalence of current cigarette smoking among adults, and policies and attitudes about secondhand smoke—United States, 2000. *Morbidity and Mortality Weekly Report.* 2001b;50(49):1101–6.

Centers for Disease Control and Prevention. *Second National Report on Human Exposure to Environmental Chemicals.* Atlanta: U.S. Department of Health and Human Services, Centers for Disease Control and Prevention, National Center for Environmental Health, 2003. NCEH Publication No. 02-0716.

Centers for Disease Control and Prevention. *Third National Report on Human Exposure to Environmental Chemicals.* Atlanta: U.S. Department of Health and Human Services, Centers for Disease Control and Prevention, National Center for Environmental Health, 2005. NCEH Publication No.05-0570.

Coghlin J, Gann PH, Hammond SK, Skipper PL, Taghizadeh K, Paul M. 4-Aminobiphenyl hemo globin adducts in fetuses exposed to the tobacco smoke carcinogen in utero. *Journal of the National Cancer Institute.* 1991;83(4):274–80.

Coghlin J, Hammond SK, Gann PH. Development of epidemiologic tools for measuring environmental tobacco smoke exposure. *American Journal of Epidemiology.* 1989;130(4):696–704.

Coultas DB, Howard CA, Peake GT, Skipper BJ, Samet JM. Salivary cotinine levels and involuntary tobacco smoke exposure in children and adults in New Mexico. *American Review of Respiratory Disease.* 1987;136(2):305–9.

Ebrahim SH, Floyd RL, Merritt RK II, Decoufle P, Holtzman D. Trends in pregnancy-related smoking rates in the United States, 1987–1996. *Journal of the American Medical Association.* 2000;283(3):361–6.

Emmons KM, Hammond SK, Fava JL, Velicer WF, Evans JL, Monroe AD. A randomized trial to reduce passive smoke exposure in low-income households with young children. *Pediatrics.* 2001;108(1):18–24.

Ferris BG Jr, Ware JH, Berkey CS, Dockery DW, Spiro A III, Speizer FE. Effects of passive smoking on health of children. *Environmental Health Perspectives.* 1985;62:289–95.

Ford RP, Tappin DM, Schluter PJ, Wild CJ. Smoking during pregnancy: how reliable are maternal self reports in New Zealand? *Journal of Epidemiology and Community Health.* 1997;51(3):246–51.

Gilpin EA, Emery SL, Farkas AJ, Distefan JM, White MM, Pierce JP. *The California Tobacco Control Program: A Decade of Progress, Results from the California Tobacco Surveys, 1990–1999.* La Jolla (CA): Univer sity of California, San Diego, 2001.

Giovino GA, Henningfield JE, Tomar SL, Esc obedo LG, Slade J. Epidemiology of tobacco use and dependence [review]. *Epidemiologic Reviews.* 1995;17(1):48–65.

Greenberg RA, Bauman KE, Glover LH, Strecher VJ, Kleinbaum DG, Haley NJ, Stedman HC, Fowler MG, Loda FA. Ecology of passive smoking by young infants. *Journal of Pediatrics.* 1989;114(5):774–80.

Haddow JE, Knight GJ, Palomaki GE, Kloza EM, Wald NJ. Cigarette consumption and serum cotinine in relation to birthweight. *British Journal of Obstetrics and Gynaecology.* 1987;94(7):678–81.

Hammond SK. Exposure of U.S. workers to envi ronmental tobacco smoke [review]. *Environmental Health Perspectives.* 1999;107(Suppl 2) :329–40.

Hammond SK, Coghlin J, Gann PH, Paul M, Taghiza deh K, Skipper PL, Tannenbaum SR. Relationship between environmental tobacco smoke exposure and carcinogen–hemoglobin adduct levels in non smokers. *Journal of the National Cancer Institute.* 1993;85(6):474–8.

Hammond SK, Perrino C. Passive smoking in non smoking sections of 71 Indiana restaurants [abstract]. *Epidemiology.* 2002;13(4):S145–S146.

Jaakkola MS, Jaakkola JJ. Assessment of exposure to environmental tobacco smoke. *European Respiratory Journal.* 1997;10(10):2384–97.

Jaakkola MS, Samet JM. Summary: workshop on health risks attributable to ETS exposure in the workplace. *Environmental Health Perspectives.* 1999;107(Suppl 6):823–8.

Jarvis MJ, Foulds J, Feyerabend C. Exposure to passive smoking among bar staff. *British Journal of Addiction.* 1992;87(1):111–3.

Jarvis MJ, Goddard E, Higgins V, Feyerabend C, Bry ant A, Cook DG. Children's exposure to passive smoking in England since the 1980s: cotinine evi dence from population surveys. *British Medical Journal.* 2000;321(7257):343–5.

Jarvis MJ, Tunstall-Pedoe H, Feyerabend C, Vesey C, Saloojee Y. Comparison of tests used to distinguish smokers from nonsmokers. *American Journal of Public Health.* 1987;77(11):1435–8.

Jenkins RA, Counts RW. Personal exposure to envi ronmental tobacco smoke: salivary cotinine, air borne nicotine, and nonsmoker misclassification. *Journal of Exposure Analysis and Environmental Epidemiology.* 1999;9(4):352–63.

Jenkins RA, Guerin MR, Tomkins BA. *The Chemistry of Environmental Tobacco Smoke: Composition and Measurement.* 2nd ed. Boca Raton (FL): Lewis, 2000.

Jenkins RA, Palausky A, Counts RW, Bayne CK, Dindal AB, Guerin MR. Exposure to environmental tobacco smoke in sixteen cities in the United States as determined by personal breathing zone air sam pling. *Journal of Exposure Analysis and Environmental Epidemiology.* 1996a;6(4):473–502.

Jenkins RA, Palausky MA, Counts RW, Guerin MR, Dindal AB, Bayne CK. Determination of per sonal exposure of non-smokers to environmental tobacco smoke in the United States. *Lung Cancer.* 1996b;14(Suppl 1):S195–S213.

Kegler MC, Malcoe LH. Smoking restrictions in the home and car among rural Native American and white families with young children. *Preventive Medicine.* 2002;35(4):334–42.

King G, Strouse R, Hovey DA, Zehe L. Cigarette smok ing in Connecticut: home and workplace exposure. *Connecticut Medicine.* 1998;62(9):531–9.

Klepeis NE. An introduction to the indirect exposure assessment approach: modeling human exposure using microenvironmental measurements and the recent National Human Activity Pattern Survey. *Environmental Health Perspectives.* 1999;107(Suppl 2):365–74.

Klepeis NE, Nelson WC, Ott WR, Robinson JP, Tsang AM, Switzer P, Behar JV, Hern SC, Engelmann WH. The National Human Activity Pattern Survey (NHAPS): a resource for assessing exposure to envi ronmental pollutants. *Journal of Exposure Analysis and Environmental Epidemiology.* 2001;11(3):231–52.

Kottke TE, Aase LA, Brandel CL, Brekke MJ, Brekke LN, DeBoer SW, Hoffman RS, Menzel PA, Thomas RJ. Attitudes of Olmsted County, Minnesota, resi dents about tobacco smoke in restaurants and bars. *Mayo Clinic Proceedings* 2001;76(2):134–7.

Lambert WE, Samet JM, Spengler JD. Environmental tobacco smoke concentrations in no-smoking and smoking sections of restaurants. *American Journal of Public Health.* 1993;83(9):1339–41.

Leaderer BP, Hammond SK. Evaluation of vapor- phase nicotine and respirable suspended particle mass as markers for environmental tobacco smoke. *Environmental Science and Technology.* 1991;25(4):770–7.

Lebowitz MD, Burrows B. Respiratory symptoms related to smoking habits of family adults. *Chest.* 1976;69(1):48–50.

Maier WC, Arrighi HM, Morray B, Llewellyn C, Red ding GJ. Indoor risk factors for asthma and wheez ing among Seattle school children. *Environmental Health Perspectives.* 1997;105(2):208–14.

Manning SC, Wasserman RL, Silver R, Phillips DL. Results of endoscopic sinus surgery in pediat ric patients with chronic sinusitis and asthma. *Archives of Otolaryngology—Head and Neck Surgery.* 1994;120(10):1142–5.

Mannino DM, Caraballo R, Benowitz N, Repace J. Pre dictors of cotinine levels in US children: data from the Third National Health and Nutrition Examina tion Survey. *Chest.* 2001;120(3):718–24.

Mannino DM, Siegel M, Husten C, Rose D, Etzel R. Environmental tobacco smoke exposure and health effects in children: results from the 1991 National Health Interview Survey. *Tobacco Control.* 1996;5(1):13–8.

Mannino DM, Siegel M, Rose D, Nkuchia J, Etzel R. Environmental tobacco smoke exposure in the home and worksite and health effects in adults: results from the 1991 National Health Interview Survey. *Tobacco Control.* 1997;6(4):296–305.

Marbury MC, Hammond SK, Haley NJ. Measuring exposure to environmental tobacco smoke in stud ies of acute health effects. *American Journal of Epidemiology.* 1993;137(10):1089–97.

Margolis PA, Keyes LL, Greenberg RA, Bauman KE, LaVange LM. Urinary cotinine and parent history (questionnaire) as indicators of passive smok ing and predictors of lower respiratory illness in infants. *Pediatric Pulmonology.* 1997;23(6):417–23.

Maskarinec MP, Jenkins RA, Counts RW, Dindal AB. Determination of exposure to environmental tobacco smoke in restaurant and tavern workers in one US city. *Journal of Exposure Analysis and Environmental Epidemiology.* 2000;10(1):36–49.

McMillen RC, Winickoff JP, Klein JD, Weitzman M. US adult attitudes and practices regarding smoking restrictions and child exposure to environmental tobacco smoke: changes in the social climate from 2000–2001. *Pediatrics.* 2003;112(1 Pt 1):E55–E60.

Muramatsu M, Umemura S, Okada T, Tomita H. Estimation of personal exposure to tobacco smoke with a newly developed nicotine personal monitor. *Environmental Research.* 1984;35(1):218–27.

Norman GJ, Ribisl KM, Howard-Pitney B, Howard KA. Smoking bans in the home and car: do those who really need them have them? *Preventive Medicine.* 1999;29(6 Pt 1):581–9.

O'Connor TZ, Holford TR, Leaderer BP, Hammond SK, Bracken MB. Measurement of exposure to environmental tobacco smoke in pregnant women. *American Journal of Epidemiology.* 1995;142(12):1315–21.

Overpeck MD, Moss AJ. Children's exposure to envi ronmental cigarette smoke before and after birth: health of our nation's children, United States, 1988. *Advances in Data.* 1991;(202):1–11.

Phillips K, Bentley MC, Abrar M, Howard DA, Cook J. Low level saliva cotinine determination and its application as a biomarker for environmental tobacco smoke exposure. *Human and Experimental Toxicology.* 1999a;18(4):291–6.

Phillips K, Bentley MC, Howard DA, Alván G. Assess ment of air quality in Stockholm by personal moni toring of nonsmokers for respirable suspended particles and environmental tobacco smoke. *Scandinavian Journal of Work, Environment and Health.* 1996;22(Suppl 1):1–24.

Phillips K, Bentley MC, Howard DA, Alván G. Assess ment of air quality in Paris by personal monitoring of nonsmokers for respirable suspended particles and environmental tobacco smoke. *Envronment International.* 1998a;24(4):405–25.

Phillips K, Bentley MC, Howard DA, Alván G. Assess ment of environmental tobacco smoke and respira ble suspended particle exposures for nonsmokers in Kuala Lumpur using personal monitoring. *Journal of Exposure Analysis and Environmental Epidemiology.* 1998b;8(4):519–42.

Phillips K, Bentley MC, Howard DA, Alván G. Assess ment of environmental tobacco smoke and respirable suspended particle exposures for nonsmokers in Prague using personal monitoring. *International Archives of Occupational and Environmental Health.* 1998c;71(6):379–90.

Phillips K, Bentley MC, Howard DA, Alván G, Huici A. Assessment of air quality in Barcelona by per sonal monitoring of nonsmokers for respirable suspended particles and environmental tobacco smoke. *Environment International.* 1997a;23(2):173–96.

Phillips K, Howard DA, Bentley MC, Alván G. Assess ment of air quality in Turin by personal monitoring of nonsmokers for respirable suspended particles and environmental tobacco smoke. *Environment International.* 1997b; 23(6):851–71.

Phillips K, Howard DA, Bentley MC, Alván G. Assess ment by personal monitoring of respirable sus pended particles and environmental tobacco smoke exposure for nonsmokers in Sydney, Australia. *Indoor and Built Environment.* 1998d;7(4):188–203.

Phillips K, Howard DA, Bentley MC, Alván G. Assess ment of environmental tobacco smoke and respira ble suspended particle exposures for nonsmokers in Basel by personal monitoring. *Atmospheric Environment.* 1999b;33(12):1889–904.

Phillips K, Howard DA, Bentley MC, Alván G. Assess ment of environmental tobacco smoke and respira ble suspended particle exposures for nonsmokers in Hong Kong using personal monitoring. *Environment International.* 1998e;24(8):851–70.

Phillips K, Howard DA, Bentley MC, Alván G. Assess ment of environmental tobacco smoke and respira ble suspended particle exposures for nonsmokers in Lisbon by personal monitoring. *Environment International.* 1998f;24(3):301–24.

Phillips K, Howard DA, Bentley MC, Alván G. Envi ronmental tobacco smoke and respirable suspended particle exposures for nonsmokers in Beijing. *Indoor and Built Environment.* 1998g;7(5–6):254–69.

Phillips K, Howard DA, Bentley MC, Alván G. Mea sured exposures by personal monitoring for respira ble suspended particles and environmental tobacco smoke of housewives and office workers resident in Bremen, Germany. *International Archives of Occupational and Environmental Health.* 1998h;71(3):201–12.

Pierce JP, Gilpin EA, Emery SL, Farkas AJ, Zhu SH, Choi WS, Berry CC, Distefan JM, White MM, Sor ato S, Navarro A. *Tobacco Control in California: Who's Winning the War? An Evaluation of the Tobacco Control Program, 1989–1996.* La Jolla (CA): University of California, San Diego, 1998.

Pirkle JL, Bernert JT, Caudill SP, Sosnoff CS, Pechacek TF. Trends in the exposure of nonsmokers in the U.S. population to secondhand smoke: 1988–2002. *Environmental Health Perspectives.* 2006;114(6):853–8.

Pirkle JL, Flegal KM, Bernert JT, Brody DJ, Etzel RA, Maurer KR. Exposure of the US population to environmental tobacco smoke: the Third National Health and Nutrition Examination Survey, 1988 to 1991. *Journal of the American Medical Association.* 1996;275(16):1233–40.

Samet JM, Wang SS. Environmental tobacco smoke. In: Lippman M, editor. *Environmental Toxicants: Human Exposures and Their Health Effects.* 2nd ed. New York: John Wiley and Sons, 2000:319–75.

Schilling RS, Letai AD, Hui SL, Beck GJ, Schoenberg JB, Bouhuys A. Lung function, respiratory disease, and smoking in families. *American Journal of Epidemiology.* 1977;106(4):274–83.

Schuster MA, Franke T, Pham CB. Smoking patterns of household members and visitors in homes with children in the United States. *Archives of Pediatrics and Adolescent Medicine.* 2002;156(11):1094–100.

Shopland DR, Gerlach KK, Burns DM, Hartman AM, Gibson JT. State-specific trends in smoke-free workplace policy coverage: the current popula tion survey tobacco use supplement, 1993 to 1999. *Journal of Occupational and Environmental Medicine.* 2001;43(8):680–6.

Shopland DR, Hartman AM, Gibson JT, Mueller MD, Kessler LG, Lynn WR. Cigarette smoking among U.S. adults by state and region: estimates from the current population survey. *Journal of the National Cancer Institute.* 1996;88(23):1748–58.

Siegel M, Albers AB, Cheng DM, Biener L, Rigotti NA. Effect of local restaurant smoking regulations on environmental tobacco smoke exposure among youths. *American Journal of Public Health.* 2004;94(2):321–5.

Skeer M, Siegel M. The descriptive epidemiology of local restaurant smoking regulations in Massachusetts: an analysis of the protection of restaurant customers and workers. *Tobacco Control.* 2003;12(2):221–6.

Soliman S, Pollack HA, Warner KE. Decrease in the prevalence of environmental tobacco smoke exposure in the home during the 1990s in families with children. *American Journal of Public Health.* 2004;94(2):314–20.

U.S. Department of Health and Human Services. *The Health Consequences of Involuntary Smoking. A Report of the Surgeon General.* Rockville (MD): U.S. Department of Health and Human Services, Public Health Service, Centers for Disease Control, Center for Health Promotion and Education, Office on Smoking and Health, 1986. DHHS Publication No. (CDC) 87-8398.

Windsor RA, Lowe JB, Perkins LL, Smith-Yoder D, Artz L, Crawford M, Amburgy K, Boyd NRF Jr. Health education for pregnant smokers: its behavioral impact and cost benefit. *American Journal of Public Health.* 1993;83(2):201–6.

In: Children and Secondhand Smoke Exposure
Editor: J. R. Harrington

ISBN: 978-1-60692-587-4
© 2009 Nova Science Publishers, Inc.

Chapter 3

EXCERPTS FROM CHAPTER 5. REPRODUCTIVE AND DEVELOPMENTAL EFFECTS FROM EXPOSURE TO SECONDHAND SMOKE

INTRODUCTION

This chapter concerns adverse effects on repro duction, infants, and child development from exposure to secondhand smoke. Previous Surgeon General's reports have not comprehensively addressed the relationship between secondhand smoke exposure and reproductive outcomes, infant mortality, or child development. The 2001 Surgeon General's report (*Women and Smoking*) did summarize the literature on developmental and reproductive outcomes in relation to secondhand smoke exposure, focusing on the spe cific outcomes of fertility and fecundity, fetal growth and birth weight, fetal loss and neonatal mortality, and congenital malformations (U.S. Department of Health and Human Services [USDHHS] 2001).

The effects of active smoking by the mother during pregnancy were comprehensively reviewed in the 2004 report (USDHHS 2004). This new report reviews the possible effects of secondhand smoke exposure on reproductive and developmental outcomes, incor porates the substantial amount of evidence that has emerged since the 1986 Surgeon General's report (*The Health Consequences of Involuntary Smoking*, USDHHS 1986), and expands upon the 2001 report.

The epidemiologic evidence is reviewed in detail in the full report. Therefore, it is not included in this Excerpt. The full report may be accessed at http://www.surgeongeneral.gov/library/secondhandsmoke/report.

CONCLUSIONS OF PREVIOUS SURGEON GENERAL'S REPORTS AND OTHER RELEVANT REPORTS

The early literature on secondhand smoke exposure and child health focused on adverse respiratory effects. Initial relevant reports were first published in the 1960s (Cameron et al. 1969), followed by larger studies in the 1970s (Colley 1974; Colley et al. 1974). The first summary report to comprehensively address reproductive and perinatal effects of secondhand smoke exposure was prepared by the California Environmental Protection Agency and released in 1997 (National Cancer Institute [NCI] 1999). These topics were also addressed by a number of other agencies and groups, including the United Kingdom Department of Health (1998), the World Health Organization (WHO 1999), and the University of Toronto (2001). Table 5.1 in the full report summarizes the conclusions for reproductive and perinatal outcomes from these reports.

LITERATURE SEARCH METHODS

The authors identified most of the literature on secondhand smoke exposure and adverse reproductive and perinatal effects through a systematic search of the National Library of Medicine's indexed journals, which date back to 1966. The relevant Medical Subject Headings (MeSH) terms and text terms were used to search PubMed. Text terms were used because many of the relevant MeSH terms were not introduced into the PubMed key wording scheme until some time after 1966. For example, the MeSH term "Tobacco Smoke Pollution" was not introduced until 1982. The following text terms were also used in the search for articles: environmental, tobacco, smoke, secondhand smoke, paternal smoking, and passive smoking. By combining these text terms and MeSH terms using "or" as the Boolean connector, nearly 4,500 citations were identified. The authors also used this strategy to identify relevant research on outcomes. The results of each outcome-relevant search were then combined with the secondhand smoke-relevant search using "and" as the Boolean connector. These citations were imported into a database. Using title and abstract information, the authors selected the relevant

CRITICAL EXPOSURE PERIODS FOR REPRODUCTIVE AND DEVELOPMENT EFFECTS

Assessing exposures to secondhand smoke in studies of fertility, fetal development, infant development, and child health and development is complex. For each of the three biologically relevant periods— preconception, pregnancy, and postdelivery—a number of potentially different biologic mechanisms of injury exist from exposure to secondhand smoke. Even within the nine months of pregnancy, vulnerability to the effects of secondhand smoke may change, reflecting differing mechanisms of injury as fetal organs develop and the fetus grows. Moreover, there are multiple environments where the woman or child is exposed to secondhand smoke (e.g., workplace, home, and day care), as well as multiple sources of secondhand smoke exposure for each of these environments (e.g., household members, day care providers, and coworkers). Finally, because of the potential impact of active maternal smoking (USDHHS 2004), active smoking before and during pregnancy needs to be taken into account when assessing the potential independent effects of exposure to secondhand smoke. Maternal smoking has well-characterized adverse effects for several outcomes, such as fertility, sudden infant death syndrome (SIDS), and child growth and development. Thus, the effects of exposure to secondhand smoke may be confounded by those of maternal smoking.

Secondhand smoke exposure may have adverse effects potentially throughout the reproductive and developmental processes. During the preconception period, maternal exposure to secondhand smoke can potentially affect female fertility by altering the balance of hormones that affect oocyte production, including growth hormone, cortisol, luteinizing hormones, and prolactin (Mattison 1982; Daling et al. 1987; Mattison and Thomford 1987), or by reducing motility in the female reproductive tract (Mattison 1982; Daling et al. 1987). However, separating the potential effect of secondhand smoke exposure on the mother's reproductive process and the effect of active paternal smoking on the father's reproductive process is very difficult. Although the evidence is mixed, active smoking has been shown to affect sperm morphology, motility, and concentration (Rosenberg 1987; USDHHS 2004). Cigarette smoke may also lead to infertility through a combined effect of decreased sperm motility with active paternal smoking and decreased tubal patency with active maternal smoking and secondhand smoke exposure.

During pregnancy, maternal exposure to secondhand smoke could potentially affect the pregnancy by increasing the risk for spontaneous abortion or by interfering with the developing fetus through growth restrictions or congenital malformations (NCI 1999; WHO 1999). During gestation, windows of susceptibility exist when the developing embryo or fetus is vulnerable to various intrauterine conditions or exposures. Organogenesis occurs mainly during the embryonic period (weeks three through eight of gestation), which is also the time when major malformations are most likely to develop. During weeks 9 through 38 of gestation, susceptibility decreases and insults are more likely to lead to minor malformations or functional defects (Sadler 1990).

Finally, secondhand smoke exposure in the postpartum period could affect the developing infant and child, resulting in a number of adverse health outcomes. Given the developmental processes in progress, infants and children are considered to be more vulnerable to the effects of environmental exposures than are adults (Goldman 1995; Dempsey et al. 2000). Mechanisms that could lead to compromised physical and cognitive development as a result of exposure to secondhand smoke may be similar to the processes that affect fetal development, such as hypoxia (USDHHS 1990; Lambers and Clark 1996). One review of the impact of prenatal exposure to nicotine summarized numerous animal studies that demonstrated the effects of nicotine on cognitive processes among exposed rats and guinea pigs, such as impeded learning abilities or increased attention or memory deficits (Ernst et al. 2001). In animal and human studies, prenatal nicotine exposure affected aspects of neural functioning such as the activation of neurotransmitter systems, which may lead to permanent alterations in the developing brain through changes in gene expression. The proposed consequences of altered gene expression included disturbances in neuronal pathfinding and in cell regulation and differentiation (Ernst et al. 2001). Other animal studies have shown that newborn rats exposed to sidestream smoke have reduced DNA and protein concentrations in the brain (Gospe et al. 1996). Ideally, researchers should have information on secondhand smoke exposures for all relevant periods that relate to the outcome under study, because different physiologic processes may be affected across developmental periods. However, this information is frequently unavailable in a particular study.

Secondhand smoke exposures most commonly occur in the home or workplace, and exposures in public places tend to be more sporadic. Recent exposure assessment and monitoring studies have shown that the home tends to be a greater source of secondhand smoke exposure than the workplace (Emmons et al. 1994; Pirkle et al. 1996; Hammond 1999), particularly since workplace smoking bans have become more restrictive (Marcus et al. 1992) (Chapter 3, Assess ment of Exposure to Secondhand Smoke, in the full report, and Chapter 4, Prevalence of Exposure to Secondhand Smoke). In the home, the major sources of exposures to secondhand smoke have been smoking by the spouse or partner and other household mem bers. Paternal smoking has been the most commonly measured source of secondhand smoke in the home (USDHHS 1986), and paternal smoking status tends to be constant across the three developmental periods: preconception, prenatal, and postnatal (USDHHS 1986). Although many studies have not considered smoking in the home by other household members, some studies have documented that such smok ing could be a significant source of secondhand smoke exposure for women (Pattishall et al. 1985; Rebagliato et al. 1995; Pirkle et al. 1996; Ownby et al. 2000; Kaufman et al. 2002). Studies on workplace exposure have focused on whether or not the person was exposed, but less attention has been paid to quan tifying the exposure (Misra and Nguyen 1999).

FERTILITY

Biologic Basis

Infertility is commonly defined as a failure to conceive after 12 months of unprotected intercourse. Infertility should not be confused with fecundabil ity, which is defined as the probability of conception during one menstrual cycle and measured by time to pregnancy. Thus, low fecundability is delayed con ception. The biologic plausibility that secondhand smoke exposure affects human fertility and fecund- ability is supported by both animal and human stud ies of active smoking, which include exposure to the same materials as involuntary smoking. In animal studies, numerous investigators have demonstrated the biologic effects of nicotine in disrupting oviduct function (Neri and Marcus 1972; Ruckebusch 1975) and in delaying blastocyst formation and implanta tion (Yoshinaga et al. 1979). Investigations of assisted reproduction among humans who actively smoke have also provided information on possible mecha nisms of infertility and delayed conception from sec ondhand smoke exposure. Several studies of assisted reproductive techniques have suggested that active maternal smoking reduces the estradiol level in fol licular fluid (Elenbogen et al. 1991; Van Voorhis et al. 1992), impedes ovulation induction (Van Voorhis et al. 1992; Chung et al. 1997), reduces the fertilization rate (Elenbogen et al. 1991; Rosevear et al. 1992), and retards the embryo cleavage rate (dose-dependent) (Hughes et al. 1992). Metabolites of cigarette smoke have been measured in the follicular fluid of active smokers at assisted reproduction clinics (Trapp et al. 1986; Weiss and Eckert 1989; Rosevear et al. 1992) and in the cervical mucus of active smokers in a cervical cancer study (Sasson et al. 1985).

Together, the evidence from studies of biologic mechanisms and the findings of numerous epidemi ologic studies have led to the conclusion that active maternal smoking causes reduced fertility. An early review by Stillman and colleagues (1986) of studies of natural reproduction in addition to the two most recent Surgeon General's reports (USDHHS 2001, 2004) sup port this conclusion of a causal association, and find ings of meta-analyses have provided estimates of the magnitude of the effect of maternal smoking on fertil ity. Hughes and Brennan (1996) combined the results of seven studies on in vitro fertilization with gamete intrafallopian transfer. Comparing smokers and non smokers, the researchers obtained a combined odds ratio (OR) for conception of 0.57 (95 percent confi dence interval [CI], 0.42–0.78). Similarly, Augood and colleagues (1998) pooled nine studies that compared smokers with nonsmokers and found a combined OR of 0.66 (95 percent CI, 0.49–0.88) for the number of pregnancies per cycle of in vitro fertilization. In their meta-analysis of 12 studies, Augood and colleagues (1998) compared smokers with nonsmokers and found that the overall OR for infertility was 1.60 (95 percent CI, 1.34–1.91). Several investigators found a dose- response trend between the level of active maternal smoking and decreased fertility (Baird and Wilcox 1985; Suonio et al. 1990; Laurent et al. 1992).

Although active paternal smoking could also play a role in infertility by affecting sperm quality, the 2004 Surgeon General's report found conflict ing evidence on active smoking and sperm quality (USDHHS 2004). In another review, investigators per formed a meta-analysis of 20 study populations (from 18 published papers) on cigarette smoking and sperm density and found a weighted estimated reduction of 13 percent in sperm density (95 percent CI, 8.0–17.1) among smokers compared with nonsmokers (Vine et al. 1994). The epidemiologic studies that have exam ined the effect of active paternal smoking on fertility are not as consistent in their findings as the studies that have investigated active maternal smoking and fertility (Underwood et al. 1967; Tokuhata 1968; Baird and Wilcox 1985; de Mouzon et al. 1988; Dunphy et al. 1991; Pattinson et al. 1991; Hughes et al. 1992; Rowlands et al. 1992; Bolumar et al. 1996; Hull et al. 2000). One review concluded that paternal smoking had no effect on fertility (Hughes and Brennan 1996).

Several studies that were conducted in repro ductive clinics measured tobacco smoke biomarkers in nonsmoking men and women exposed to second hand smoke. Cotinine was measurable in follicular fluid, with measurements related to dose (Zenzes et al. 1996), and benzo[*a*]pyrene adducts were found in ovarian cells (Zenzes et al. 1998). Both nicotine and cotinine were measured in semen of nonsmoking, secondhand smoke-exposed men attending a clinic specializing in infertility (Pacifici et al. 1995).

Evidence Synthesis

The observational evidence is quite limited. The four studies that directly address maternal second hand smoke exposure and fertility differ substantially in study design and methods. For example, Chung and colleagues (1997) investigated patients who were attending a clinic for fertility-related problems and examined the success rate of assisted reproduction. Hull and colleagues (2000), on the other hand, included pregnant women and examined delayed natural conception. In the former study, the investigators did not account for potential confounders and obtained retrospective information about exposure to secondhand smoke from telephone interviews (Chung et al. 1997). Hull and colleagues (2000) relied on a self-administered questionnaire to ascertain exposure information during pregnancy, and used potential confounders in the analysis such as parental age, body mass index, and alcohol consumption. The evidence from this larger study on natural conception is consistent with the biologic framework established by the studies on active maternal smoking and fertility (Hull et al. 2000).

Conclusion

1. The evidence is inadequate to infer the presence or absence of a causal relationship between maternal exposure to secondhand smoke and female fertility or fecundability. No data were found on paternal exposure to secondhand smoke and male fertility or fecundability.

Implications

As exposure of women of reproductive age to secondhand smoke continues, this topic needs further rigorous investigation. In particular, the frequency and extent of current exposures should be characterized. Further epidemiologic studies also merit consideration.

PREGNANCY (SPONTANEOUS ABORTION AND PERINATAL DEATH)

Biologic Basis

Fetal loss or spontaneous abortion is defined as the involuntary termination of an intrauterine pregnancy before 20 weeks of gestation (Anderson et al. 1998). Because most early fetal losses are underreported and unrecognized, spontaneous abortions are extremely difficult to study. Twenty to 40 percent of all pregnancies may terminate too early to be recognized or confirmed (Wilcox et al. 1988; Eskenazi et al. 1995). Furthermore, the etiology of spontaneous abortion is multifactorial and not fully understood. Some early miscarriages result from chromosomal abnormalities in the developing embryo; others are related to fac tors associated with maternal age, with the pregnancy itself, or to other types of exposures (e.g., occupational exposure, alcohol consumption, or fever). Moreover, relatively few animal studies have been conducted to gain an understanding of how exposure to sidestream smoke may affect the processes of spontaneous abor tion (NCI 1999). In one study of sea urchins, investi gators noted that exposure to nicotine prevented the cortical granule reaction, which typically prevents the entry of additional sperm into the egg once fer tilization has occurred (Longo and Anderson 1970). If this same process occurs in the human fertilized ovum as a result of nicotine exposure, this may be a mechanism by which abnormalities in the develop ing embryo result in spontaneous abortions (Longo and Anderson 1970; Mattison et al. 1989). Several tobacco components and metabolites are potentially toxic to the developing fetus, including lead, nicotine, cotinine, cyanide, cadmium, carbon monoxide (CO), and polycyclic aromatic hydrocarbons (Lambers and Clark 1996; Werler 1997). Finally, with regard to active smoking and spontaneous abortion, many studies have reported a greater increase in risk for smokers than for nonsmokers, and some studies have demon strated dose-response relationships (USDHHS 2004).

Evidence Synthesis

The few studies that have examined the rela tionship between involuntary smoking and sponta neous abortion have inconsistent findings. Although some studies reported an increased risk for spontane ous abortion among women exposed to secondhand smoke at work or at home, many found no association.

However, for the studies that showed no associations, the study samples may have lacked adequate statistical power.

Three studies examined secondhand smoke exposures among women who were nonsmokers. Koo and colleagues (1988) examined rates of miscarriage among 136 nonsmoking wives who were part of a larger study on cancer. These 136 women were the controls in this study, which ascertained lifetime smoking histories of the husbands and reproductive histories of the wives. Social and demographic factors differed between families with smoking and nonsmoking husbands. The crude OR for more than two miscarriages among wives with husbands who smoked was 1.81 (95 percent CI, 0.85–3.85) (adjusted ORs were not reported). Ahlborg and Bodin (1991) reported on nonsmoking women who were exposed to secondhand smoke at home. Two estimates were provided, one for first trimester losses (OR = 0.96 [95 percent CI, 0.50–1.86]) and for one second or third trimester losses (OR = 1.06 [95 percent CI, 0.55–2.05]). Windham and colleagues (1999b) reported adjusted ORs for paternal smoking among women who were nonsmokers. When maternal age, prior spontaneous abortion, alcohol and caffeine consumption, and gestational age at initial interviews were taken into account, the investigators obtained an OR of 1.15 (95 percent CI, 0.86–1.55) for secondhand smoke exposure at home. The pooled estimate from these three studies (with the two estimates from Ahlborg and Bodin [1991] included separately) for secondhand smoke exposure in the home or from fathers who smoked and who were married to nonsmoking women was 1.18 (95 percent CI, 0.92–1.44).

Future studies not only need to ensure an adequate sample size, but they should give particular attention to the difficult issues of confounding and to accurate estimates of secondhand smoke exposures in the workplace and in the home.

CONCLUSION

1. The evidence is inadequate to infer the presence or absence of a causal relationship between maternal exposure to secondhand smoke during pregnancy and spontaneous abortion.

Implications

As for other outcomes that have very few studies, further research is warranted (see "Overall Implications" later in this chapter).

INFANT DEATHS

Infant mortality is defined as the death of a live-born infant within 364 days of birth. Many of the major causes of infant deaths, such as low birth weight (LBW), preterm delivery, and SIDS, are also associated with exposure to tobacco smoke during and after pregnancy. The biologic mechanisms by which secondhand smoke exposure leads to these particular outcomes are discussed in other parts of this chapter and will not be discussed here. In 2002, the infant mortality rate for infants of smokers (11.1 percent) was 68 percent higher than the rate for infants of nonsmokers (6.6 percent) (Mathews et al. 2004). For each race and Hispanic-origin group, the infant mortality rate among infants of smokers was higher compared with the rate among infants of nonsmokers.

Evidence Synthesis

Only two studies examined the relationship of involuntary smoking with neonatal mortality. Both studies reported associations of secondhand smoke exposure from paternal smoking with neonatal mortality. There is significantly more literature on active smoking by the mother during pregnancy and neonatal outcome. Although the strength of the relationship in these two studies was strong, causality cannot be inferred because of the small number of studies and because of inadequate controls for potential confounders.

Conclusion

1. The evidence is inadequate to infer the presence or absence of a causal relationship between exposure to secondhand smoke and neonatal mortality.

Implications

In addition to the consistent relationship demonstrated between exposure to secondhand smoke and neonatal mortality, numerous studies have reported significant associations between active maternal smoking during pregnancy and infant mortality. Thus, the association of secondhand smoke exposure during pregnancy and infant mortality warrants further investigation. Moreover, the data cited were from older studies, and smoking patterns and levels of secondhand smoke exposure may have changed since the time some of the studies were conducted. To clarify the association between maternal smoking and infant mortality, more evidence is needed.

SUDDEN INFANT DEATH SYNDROME

The sudden, unexplained, unexpected death of an infant before one year of age—referred to as SIDS—has been investigated in relation to exposure of the fetus and infant to smoking by mothers and others during the preconception, prenatal, and post partum periods. The death rate attributable to SIDS has declined by more than half during the past two decades (Ponsonby et al. 2002; American Academy of Pediatrics [AAP] Task Force on SIDS 2005). SIDS has decreased dramatically because of interventions such as the "Back to Sleep" campaign implemented in the 1990s (Gibson et al. 2000; Malloy 2002; Malloy and Freeman 2004). Numerous studies have examined the association between active smoking among mothers during pregnancy and the subsequent risk of SIDS. The evidence for active smoking has demonstrated a causal association between maternal smoking during pregnancy and SIDS (Anderson and Cook 1997; United Kingdom Department of Health 1998; USDHHS 2001). The 2004 Surgeon General's report concluded that the evidence is sufficient to infer a causal relationship between SIDS and maternal smoking during and after pregnancy (USDHHS 2004). This new 2006 Surgeon General's report considers exposure of the infant to secondhand smoke from the mother, father, or others (USDHHS 2006).

Biologic Basis

Although studies have identified social and behavioral risk factors for SIDS, the biologic mecha nism or mechanisms underlying sudden, unexplained, unexpected death before one year of age are still unknown (Joad 2000; AAP Task Force on SIDS 2005). Chapter 2 (Toxicology of Secondhand Smoke) in the full report reviews the animal and human studies that provide evidence on how prenatal and postnatal exposure to nicotine and to other toxicants in tobacco smoke may affect the neuroregulation of breathing, apneic spells, and risk for sudden infant death. Exper imental data from animal models on the neurotoxic ity of prenatal and neonatal exposure to nicotine and secondhand smoke can be related to several potential causal mechanisms for SIDS, including adverse effects on brain cell development, synaptic development and function, and neurobehavioral activity (Slotkin 1998; Slotkin et al. 2001, 2006; Machaalani et al. 2005). Stick and colleagues (1996) observed newborns in the hos pital and reported reductions in respiratory function among infants of smokers compared with infants of nonsmokers. Other proposed mechanisms for post-partum reductions in respiratory function have included irritation of the airways by tobacco smoke, susceptibility to respiratory infections that increases the risk of SIDS, and a change in the ventilatory responses to hypoxia attributable to nicotine (Ander son and Cook 1997).

A diagnosis of SIDS requires supporting evi dence from an autopsy so as to exclude other causes. Thus, SIDS is a difficult outcome to study. Numer ous studies have examined the association between active smoking among mothers during pregnancy and the subsequent risk of SIDS. The evidence for active smoking has demonstrated a causal association between maternal smoking during pregnancy and SIDS (Anderson and Cook 1997; United Kingdom Department of Health 1998; USDHHS 2001, 2004).

Evidence Synthesis

The biologic evidence, especially from animal models, indicates multiple mechanisms by which exposure to secondhand smoke could cause SIDS. The evidence for secondhand smoke exposure and the risk of SIDS consistently demonstrates an association between postpartum maternal smoking and SIDS. The 1997 meta-analysis of 39 relevant studies pro duced an adjusted OR for postnatal maternal smoking of 1.94 (95 percent CI, 1.55–2.43), a level of risk that the authors concluded was almost certainly causal (Anderson and Cook 1997). Data from the four studies published since the 1997 meta-analysis add additional support for this conclusion. Nine of the thirteen stud ies in table 5.5 (see page 182 in the full report) more fully controlled for the major potential confounders (e.g., maternal smoking during pregnancy and routine sleeping position), and many controlled for a broad range of other relevant factors including maternal age, birth weight, and bed sharing. The nine studies all observed significant positive associations between postpartum maternal smoking and SIDS. Moreover, several studies demonstrated a dose-response rela tionship for secondhand smoke exposure attributable to postpartum maternal smoking, with increasing ORs for higher levels of postpartum maternal smok ing. Finally, among the studies of postnatal maternal smoking with better adjustment for confounding, the adjusted

ORs are sufficiently large, all greater than 1.5 and three of the five greater than 2.0. These ORs make it unlikely that this association is attributable to any residual confounding from unmeasured factors.

The epidemiologic evidence for secondhand smoke exposure from postpartum maternal smoking associated with the risk of SIDS is consistent and strong, and demonstrates a dose-response relationship. Evidence for secondhand smoke exposures from fathers and "other" smokers (as well as higher concentrations of nicotine and cotinine in children who die from SIDS compared with children who die of other causes) provides additional supporting evidence that secondhand smoke exposure increases the risk of SIDS. Although measures of paternal and "other" smokers in the household are not typically considered to be a comprehensive indicator of the infant's exposure to secondhand smoke, designs that can evaluate paternal smoking have the potential to more fully control for the possible confounding of maternal smoking during pregnancy. However, when considering evidence that supports an association between SIDS and paternal and "other" smokers, researchers also recognize the possible misclassification of actual infant exposures to tobacco smoke from these sources (Klonoff-Cohen et al. 1995; Dwyer et al. 1999). Despite this methodologic challenge, researchers observed an elevated OR in all nine studies of paternal smoking, ranging from 1.4 to 3.5, with many estimates around 2 or higher. Of these nine studies, five observed an elevated OR for households where the fathers smoked compared with households where neither parent smoked, and an OR of 8.5 for infants of fathers who smoked in the same room as the infant, adjusting for maternal smoking during pregnancy, routine sleeping position, and other factors. Also, out of the nine studies that examined paternal smoking, five found a statistically significant association between paternal smoking and SIDS after adjusting for maternal smoking during pregnancy. Despite the potential for misclassification bias linking paternal smoking to an actual exposure of the infant to secondhand smoke, the pooled risk estimate was 1.9 (95 percent CI, 1.01–2.80) from the five studies of paternal smoking with stronger designs that used meta-analytic approaches and random effects modeling. Finally, all of the studies of "other" smokers in the household observed an elevated OR; however, the results that adjusted for maternal smoking during pregnancy and other important confounders were more mixed. The one study with the strongest assessment of infant exposures from "other" smoking residents (i.e., live-in adults smoking in the same room as the infant) reported an OR of 4.99 (95 percent CI, 1.69–14.75), with adjustment for multiple risk factors including maternal smoking during pregnancy and routine sleeping position (Klonoff-Cohen et al. 1995).

Researchers have established prenatal maternal smoking as a major preventable risk for SIDS (USD HHS 2001, 2004; AAP Task Force on SIDS 2005). Evidence indicates that exposure of infants to sec ondhand smoke from postpartum maternal smoking has a significant additive effect on risk if the mother smoked during pregnancy. In studies that accounted for maternal smoking during pregnancy, evidence indicates that postpartum maternal smoking, particu larly in proximity to the infant, significantly increases the risk of SIDS. In addition, epidemiologic evidence indicates that postnatal exposure of infants to second hand smoke from fathers or other live-in smokers can also increase the risk of SIDS. Thus, the full range of biologic and epidemiologic data are consistent and indicate that exposure of infants to secondhand smoke causes SIDS.

Conclusion

1. The evidence is sufficient to infer a causal relationship between exposure to secondhand smoke and sudden infant death syndrome.

Implications

On the basis of the epidemiologic risk data, researchers have estimated that the population attrib utable risk of SIDS associated with postnatal exposure to secondhand smoke is about 10 percent (Cal/EPA 2005). Therefore, the evidence indicates that these exposures are one of the major preventable risk factors for SIDS, and all measures should be taken to protect infants from exposure to secondhand smoke.

There is a need for additional research to further characterize the risk of SIDS associated with prenatal and postnatal exposure to secondhand smoke, and to evaluate the relationship between maternal smoking and infant sleeping positions and bed sharing. Future research should also focus on better assessments of actual exposures of infants to secondhand smoke using biochemical assessments and/or more detailed interviews, rather than indirect assessments based on the smoking status of household adults. Because of the continuing and significant racial disparities in infant mortality from SIDS (Malloy and Freeman 2004), there is a need to study the preventable risks factors that could be involved.

PRETERM DELIVERY

Biologic Basis

Pregnancy complications, including premature labor, placenta previa, abruptio placentae, and pre mature membrane rupture may lead to preterm deliv ery (<37 completed weeks of gestation). Although the underlying mechanisms are not yet fully charac terized, maternal active smoking is associated with these pregnancy complications (U.S. Department of Health, Education, and Welfare [USDHEW] 1979b; USDHHS 1980, 2001; Andres and Day 2000). Preterm delivery is also associated with active maternal smok ing (USDHEW 1979a; USDHHS 1980, 2001; van den Berg and Oechsli 1984; Andres and Day 2000). Smok ing cessation during pregnancy appears to reduce the risk for preterm delivery (van den Berg and Oechsli 1984; Li et al. 1993; Mainous and Hueston 1994b; USDHHS 2001), placenta previa (Naeye 1980), abrup tio placentae (Naeye 1980), and premature membrane rupture (Harger et al. 1990; Williams et al. 1992); but the risk remains high for those who continue to smoke throughout pregnancy. Tobacco-specific nitrosamines and cotinine have been measured in the cervical mucus of women who were active smok ers and women who were nonsmokers (McCann et al. 1992; Prokopczyk et al. 1997). Given that active maternal smoking is associated with preterm deliv ery, this finding provided further support for the bio logic plausibility that secondhand smoke has a role in the injurious processes leading to preterm delivery. Although the biologic pathway from active maternal smoking to preterm delivery is not clear, the evidence for this association is strong enough to infer that maternal secondhand smoke exposure may also lead to preterm delivery.

Evidence Synthesis

The few studies that have evaluated the asso ciation between secondhand smoke exposure and preterm delivery have shown inconsistent findings. Of the four studies that found significant associations, two studies documented that the risk was significant only for women aged 30 years or older. Jaakkola and colleagues (2001) provided the strongest evidence for an association using hair nicotine measurements, which reduce the probability of exposure misclassifi cation. There is a biologic basis for considering this association to be causal.

Conclusion

1. The evidence is suggestive but not sufficient to infer a causal relationship between maternal exposure to secondhand smoke during pregnancy and preterm delivery.

Implications

Further research should be carried out, although studies of substantial size will be needed.

LOW BIRTH WEIGHT

Biologic Basis

Low birth weight (LBW), defined as less than 2,500 g or less than 5.5 pounds, can result from pre- term delivery or intrauterine growth retardation (IUGR), which can occur simultaneously in a preg nancy. Reduced fetal physical growth during ges tation, or IUGR, can lead to a small for gestational age (SGA) infant (10th percentile of expected birth weight for a given gestational age) that is either pre- term or full term (37 weeks of gestation), and may or may not be LBW. The established link between active maternal smoking and LBW is known to occur mainly through IUGR rather than through premature birth (Chamberlain 1975; Coleman et al. 1979; Wilcox 1993). Fetal growth is greatest during the third trimester, and studies of active smoking during pregnancy dem onstrate no reduction of infant birth weight if smok ing ceases before the third trimester (USDHHS 1990, 2004). In 2003, 12.4 percent of births among smokers were LBW (Martin et al. 2005).

A number of researchers have postulated that the limitation of fetal growth from active maternal smoking comes from reduced oxygen to the fetus, which is directly attributable to CO exposure and nicotine-induced vasoconstriction leading to reduced uterine and umbilical blood flow (USDHHS 1990, 2004; Bruner and Forouzan 1991; Rajini et al. 1994; Lambers and Clark 1996; Werler 1997; Andres and Day 2000). Studies have shown elevated nucleated red blood cell counts, a marker of fetal hypoxia, among neonates of women who actively smoked during pregnancy (Yeruchimovich et al. 1999) and among women who were exposed to secondhand smoke (Dollberg et al. 2000). Several investiga tors have also found elevated erythropoietin, the protein that stimulates red blood cell production and another indicator of hypoxia, in cord blood of newborns whose mothers had smoked during pregnancy (Jazayeri et al. 1998; Gruslin et al. 2000). Because erythropoietin does not cross the placenta, it most likely originated from the fetus. A number of researchers have also reported that the concen tration of erythropoietin is positively correlated with the concentration of cotinine measured in cord blood ($r = 0.41$, $p = 0.04$) (Gruslin et al. 2000), the number of cigarettes smoked per day by the mother ($r = 0.26$, $p < 0.0001$) (Jazayeri et al. 1998), and fetal growth retardation (r was not presented, $p < 0.01$) (Maier et al. 1993).

Studies have detected nicotine and its metabo lites perinatally in umbilical cord serum in infants born to nonsmoking mothers, and in the cervical mucus of nonsmoking women; consequently, many researchers agree that the information on active mater nal smoking is directly relevant to understanding the possible association of maternal secondhand smoke exposure and preterm delivery and LBW (USDHHS 2001). More direct evidence supports the hypothesis that maternal secondhand smoke exposure, specifi cally to nicotine, may lead to LBW through a pathway of fetal hypoxia (Çolak et al. 2002). One would expect attenuated physiologic effects from exposures to sec ondhand smoke than from active smoking based on relative dose levels, but the same biologic mechanisms of effect may apply.

Evidence Synthesis

The risk estimates for secondhand smoke expo sure and LBW have generally been small and have been consistent with the expectation that exposure to secondhand smoke should produce a smaller effect than exposure to active smoking. Most studies show a reduction in the mean birth weight and an increased risk for LBW among infants whose mothers were exposed to secondhand smoke. Across the stud ies, diverse potential confounding factors have been considered. Despite the lack of statistical significance in many of the studies, the consistencies seen in the literature have been summarized in several published reviews and have provided the strongest argument for an association between secondhand smoke and LBW. There are several plausible mechanisms by which secondhand smoke exposure could influence birth weight. Three comprehensive reviews of the literature on secondhand smoke and LBW that were published in the past decade all found a small increase in risk for LBW or SGA associated with secondhand smoke exposure (Misra and Nguyen 1999; Windham et al. 1999a; Lindbohm et al. 2002). Based on all of the studies that reported on LBW at term or SGA and sec ondhand smoke exposure, a meta-analysis provided a weighted pooled risk estimate of 1.2 (95 percent CI, 1.1–1.3) for this association (Windham et al. 1999a). Given the published review and meta-analysis by Windham and colleagues (1999a), an updated meta analysis of the relevant studies on maternal second hand smoke exposure and birth weight currently is not warranted.

Conclusion

1. The evidence is sufficient to infer a causal relationship between maternal exposure to secondhand smoke during pregnancy and a small reduction in birth weight.

Implications

Secondhand smoke exposure represents an avoidable contribution to birth weight reductions. Women, when pregnant, should not smoke or be exposed to secondhand smoke.

CONGENITAL MALFORMATIONS

Biologic Basis

Because of the direct fetal effects observed with exposure to tobacco smoke and because of the chemi cally complex and teratogenic nature of cigarette smoke, researchers have addressed the association between exposure to tobacco smoke and congenital malformations. Most of this literature has focused on active smoking during pregnancy by the mother, but a few studies have examined secondhand smoke expo sure. The etiology of most congenital malformations is not fully elaborated (Werler 1997), and no studies have been conducted to identify the mechanisms by which exposure to secondhand smoke may result in congenital malformations in humans. The few studies that have assessed the effects of sidestream smoke in animals have produced little evidence to support an association of secondhand smoke exposure and mal formations (NCI 1999). Some recent studies suggest that susceptibility to some malformations may depend in part on the presence of genes that increase suscepti bility to tobacco smoke (Wyszynski et al. 1997). Other proposed mechanisms include teratogenic effects of high concentrations of carboxyhemoglobin and nico tine, or malformations that are the result of exposure to some yet unidentified component of the tobacco plant shown to be teratogenic if ingested by animals (Seidman and Mashiach 1991).

The evidence on the relationship between mater nal smoking during pregnancy and congenital malfor mations is inconsistent. Most studies have reported no association between maternal smoking and congeni tal malformations as a whole. However, for selected malformations, particularly oral clefts, several stud ies have reported positive associations with active smoking during pregnancy by the mother (Little et al. 2004a,b; Meyer et al. 2004). In fact, recent studies on gene-environment interactions have furthered the etiologic understanding of oral clefts and the role of smoking (Hwang et al. 1995; Shaw et al. 1996; van Rooij et al. 2001, 2002; Lammer et al. 2004).

Evidence Synthesis

The evidence regarding the relationship between involuntary smoking and congenital malformations is inconsistent. The few studies that have been conducted have reported no association between involuntary smoking and specific or all congenital malformations.

Investigating congenital malformations is chal lenging because of the sample size that is necessary to study specific malformations. To date, few clues are available regarding the hypothesized biologic mecha nisms of tobacco smoke and congenital malformations. Although two studies have reported elevated rates of neural tube defects in association with involuntary smoking, this association should be examined further in future studies.

Conclusion

1. The evidence is inadequate to infer the presence or absence of a causal relationship between exposure to secondhand smoke and congenital malformations.

Implications

The topic of tobacco smoke exposure and con genital malformations merits further investigation, particularly in part because of the teratogenic nature of tobacco smoke.

COGNITIVE, BEHAVIORAL, AND PHYSICAL DEVELOPMENT

Biologic Basis

In recent years, studies have suggested that exposure to tobacco smoke during pregnancy and childhood may affect the physical and cognitive development of the growing child. Researchers who examine the effects of these exposures on childhood outcomes need to account for potential confounding factors that reflect the various correlates of second hand smoke exposure that also affect development. For example, factors that may affect physical and cognitive development include social class, parental education, the home environment as it relates to stim ulation and developmentally appropriate exposures, and pregnancy-related factors such as voluntary and involuntary smoking and alcohol and substance use. Birth weight may also be a confounding factor because it is associated with both smoking (voluntary and involuntary) and physical and cognitive develop ment. However, some researchers argue that adjust ing for birth weight may overcontrol because it may be in the causal pathway from exposure to tobacco before birth to the time when childhood outcomes are assessed (Baghurst et al. 1992).

Another methodologic challenge lies in differen tiating the effects of exposure to tobacco during and after pregnancy. This differentiation is often not pos sible because of the high correlation of tobacco smoke exposure for these two time periods. Studies with sufficient populations and detailed information on smoking status during both pregnancy and the post partum period have been able to stratify participants into exposure groups: no prenatal or postpartum expo sure, no prenatal but some postpartum exposure, and both prenatal and postpartum exposures. Other stud ies have examined the effects of secondhand smoke exposure from adults other than the mother among those children whose mothers did not smoke during pregnancy. These categories have served to partially address the timing of the exposures and, in particular, to control for exposures during pregnancy.

The mechanisms by which exposures to second hand smoke may lead to compromised physical and cognitive development have not been fully explained and may be complex. Some of the mechanisms may be similar to those proposed for maternal smoking during pregnancy, such as hypoxia or the potentially teratogenic effects of tobacco smoke (USDHHS 1990; Bruner and Forouzan 1991; Lambers and Clark 1996; Werler 1997). Studies document that components of secondhand and mainstream smoke are qualitatively similar to those of sidestream smoke, but quantitative data for doses of tobacco smoke components that reach the fetus across the placenta from active and involuntary maternal smoking have not been avail able (Slotkin 1998). This consideration is particularly important for outcomes assessed after one year of age because the child's exposure will have occurred for a period of time longer than the exposure of the fetus during the nine months of pregnancy.

For cognitive development, investigators have proposed a number of effects on central nervous system (CNS) development from smoking in general and nicotine in particular. First, the fetus may suffer from hypoxia as a result of reduced blood flow or reduced oxygen levels (USDHHS 1990; Lambers and Clark 1996). Alterations in the peripheral autonomic pathways may lead to an increased susceptibility to hypoxia-induced, short-term and long-term brain damage (Slotkin 1998). In one review of prenatal nicotine exposure, Ernst and colleagues (2001) sum marized numerous animal studies that document the impact of nicotine on cognitive processes of exposed rats and guinea pigs, such as slowed learning or increased attention or memory deficits. These inves tigators identified animal as well as human studies that have demonstrated adverse effects of nicotine exposure on neural functioning. Exposure to nicotine alters enzyme activity and thus affects brain develop ment, and alters molecular processes that affect neu rotransmitter systems and lead to permanent neural abnormalities (Ernst et al. 2001).

Cognitive Development

Evidence Synthesis
The literature cited in this discussion examined the effects of involuntary smoking on children's cognitive development. However, it is difficult to syn thesize the results of these studies because the ages of the children, the assessed exposures, and the outcomes vary across and even within studies. Moreover, some of the findings across and within studies are incon sistent. Eight of the 12 studies that examined asso ciations between involuntary smoking and children's

cognitive development reported associations between secondhand smoke exposures and reduced levels of cognitive development; these investigators had used a variety of assessments, such as performance on stan dardized tests, grade retention, or a diagnosis of men tal retardation. The use of various cognitive measures across studies precludes an assessment of consistency with specific associations. Yet the finding that second hand smoke exposure was associated with several dif ferent outcomes suggests that exposure may, indeed, impact the cognitive development of children. More studies are clearly needed; of the studies that have been conducted, there is a need for additional efforts to replicate findings.

Conclusion

1. The evidence is inadequate to infer the presence or absence of a causal relationship between exposure to secondhand smoke and cognitive functioning among children.

Implications

Further research is needed but there are complex challenges to carrying out such studies, given the need for longitudinal design and consideration of the many factors affecting cognitive functioning.

Behavioral Development

Evidence Synthesis

The evidence for an association between expo sure to secondhand smoke and behavioral problems in children is inconsistent. Because so few studies have been carried out on this topic, more studies are clearly warranted.

Conclusion

1. The evidence is inadequate to infer the presence or absence of a causal relationship between exposure to secondhand smoke and behavioral problems among children.

Implications

Further research is needed, but the same challenges remain that confront research on other effects such as cognitive functioning.

Height/Growth

Evidence Synthesis
The evidence for an association between secondhand smoke exposure and children's height/growth is mixed. Those studies that do report associations find relatively consistent deficits associated with secondhand smoke exposure. However, the magnitude of the effect is small and could reflect residual confounding.

Conclusion

1. The evidence is inadequate to infer the presence or absence of a causal relationship between exposure to secondhand smoke and children's height/growth.

Implications

The evidence suggests that any effect of secondhand smoke exposure on height is likely to be small and of little significance. Research on secondhand smoke exposure and height is complicated by the many potential confounding factors.

CHILDHOOD CANCER

Biologic Basis

Tobacco smoke contains numerous carcinogens and is a well-established cause of cancer (USDHEW 1964, 1974; USDHHS 1980, 1986; Smith et al. 1997, 2000a,b). Numerous animal studies elucidate evidence for, and mechanisms of, transplacental carcinogenesis (Rice 1979; Schuller 1984; Napalkov et al. 1989). For example, when the oncogenic compound ethylni trosourea (ENU) was administered intravenously or intraperitoneally to pregnant rabbits, the offspring developed renal and neural cancers (Stavrou et al. 1984). Monkeys are also susceptible to transplacental carcinogenesis, with offspring developing vascular and a variety of other tumors following prenatal administration of ENU to the mother (Rice et al. 1989). The strongest human evidence that transplacental car cinogenesis is biologically plausible may be the occur rence of vaginal clear-cell adenocarcinoma among young women whose mothers were prescribed dieth ylstilbesterol during pregnancy (Vessey 1989).

Limited biologic evidence suggests that invol untary exposure to cigarette smoke may also lead to transplacental carcinogenesis. Maternal secondhand smoke exposure during pregnancy, as with mater nal active smoking during pregnancy, can result in increased measurable metabolites of cigarette smoke in amniotic fluid (Andresen et al. 1982; Smith et al. 1982) and in fetal blood (Bottoms et al. 1982; Coghlin et al. 1991). For example, thiocyanate levels in fetal blood were less than 50 micromoles per liter (μmol/ L) when the mother was not exposed to secondhand smoke during pregnancy (Bottoms et al. 1982). Among mothers who were prenatally exposed to secondhand smoke, fetal blood levels of thiocyanate were as high as 90 μmol/L, and among mothers who actively smoked, the measurements were about 170 μmol/L. Notably, however, two studies that measured thio cyanate levels in umbilical cord blood found no dif ferences between secondhand smoke-exposed and unexposed nonsmoking women (Manchester and Jacoby 1981; Hauth et al. 1984). Hauth and colleagues (1984) found thiocyanate levels of 23 μmol/L in umbilical cord blood from unexposed infants of non smoking mothers and levels of 26 μmol/L in second hand smoke-exposed infants of nonsmoking mothers (defined as living and/or working with someone who smoked at least 10 cigarettes per day). Manchester and Jacoby (1981) also found similar cord blood levels of thiocyanate in unexposed (34 ± 3 μmol/L) and sec ondhand smoke-exposed (35 ± 3 μmol/L) infants of nonsmoking mothers (exposure was defined as living with someone who smoked).

Studies of maternal smoking during pregnancy found enhanced transplacental enzyme activation (Nebert et al. 1969; Manchester and Jacoby 1981) and placental DNA adducts (Everson et al. 1986, 1988; Hansen et al. 1992), and several animal studies sug gested that embryonic exposure to tobacco smoke components increased tumor rates (Mohr et al. 1975; Nicolov and Chernozemsky 1979). For example, diethylnitrosamine administered to female hamsters in the last days of pregnancy produced offspring that developed respiratory tract neoplasms in nearly 95 percent of the animals. Cigarette smoke condensate in olive oil that was used in another study of pregnant hamsters was injected intraperitoneally; it produced a variety of tumors in the offspring, including tumors of the pancreas, adrenal glands, liver, uterus, and lung (Nicolov and Chernozemsky 1979). Human studies document an increased frequency of genomic dele tions in the hypoxanthine-guanine phosphoribosyl transferase gene found in the cord blood of newborns whose mothers were exposed to secondhand smoke (compared with newborns of unexposed mothers). This finding strongly supports a carcinogenic effect of prenatal secondhand smoke exposure, particularly since these mutations are characteristic of those found in childhood leukemia and lymphoma (Finette et al. 1998). Prenatal exposure to secondhand smoke may also play a role by enhancing any effect of postnatal exposure on the development of childhood cancer (Napalkov 1973), but the potential effects of prenatal and postnatal exposures are difficult to separate given the high correlation between prenatal and postnatal parental smoking. Several studies have assessed post natal exposures by measuring cotinine and nicotine concentrations in the saliva and urine of infants. The investigators found that those infants with reported secondhand smoke exposures had significantly higher concentrations than those infants with no reported exposure in the 24 hours before measuring the concen trations (Greenberg et al. 1984; Crawford et al. 1994).

Evidence Synthesis

The strongest evidence for any childhood cancer risk from maternal secondhand smoke expo sure is specific to leukemias, lymphomas, and brain tumors, although the causal pathway may actually be through DNA damage to the father's sperm from active smoking rather than through maternal second hand smoke exposure during pregnancy. Some of the epidemiologic studies suggest a slightly increased risk in childhood cancers from prenatal and postnatal secondhand smoke exposures, but most of the stud ies were small and did not have the power to detect statistically significant associations. In addition, most of the studies lacked exposure assessments for relevant exposure periods (preconception, prenatal, and postnatal), which may also have reduced the risk estimates because of nondifferential misclassification of exposure status. Risk estimates may be inflated by recall bias, especially since interviews to assess expo sures took place up to 15 years after birth. Parents of children with cancer may be more likely to think about possible causes for their child's illness, thereby improving their recall of exposure experiences around the time of the pregnancy and birth. Parents of healthy children, however, have no particular reason to think about their exposure experiences and their recall may not be as good. Differential recall is a potential prob lem common to all case-control studies. If differential positive recall between cases and controls is present, it will inflate the risk estimate for childhood cancer.

Researchers have observed exposure-response trends for overall cancers as well as for leukemia, lymphoma, and brain tumors in a number of stud ies. Most of the studies adjusted for potentially con founding factors such as the child's date of birth, age at diagnosis, parental education level, parental age at child's birth, socioeconomic status, residence, and race by multivariate adjustment or case-control matching. Only four studies, however, considered other cancer risk factors such as maternal x-rays, drug use, and con sumption of foods containing sodium nitrite (Preston- Martin et al. 1982; Howe et al. 1989; Kuijten et al. 1990; Bunin et al. 1994). Although active maternal smoking during pregnancy does not appear to be related to childhood cancer, it was not clear in some studies whether mothers who actively smoked were excluded from the various analyses that estimated risks from paternal smoking. Thus, some of the elevated risks for cancer in their offspring from paternal smoking may have been compounded by the child's postnatal expo sure to active maternal smoking.

Conclusions

1. The evidence is suggestive but not sufficient to infer a causal relationship between prenatal and postnatal exposure to secondhand smoke and childhood cancer.
2. The evidence is inadequate to infer the presence or absence of a causal relationship between maternal exposure to secondhand smoke during pregnancy and childhood cancer.
3. The evidence is inadequate to infer the presence or absence of a causal relationship between exposure to secondhand smoke during infancy and childhood cancer.
4. The evidence is suggestive but not sufficient to infer a causal relationship between prenatal and postnatal exposure to secondhand smoke and childhood leukemias.
5. The evidence is suggestive but not sufficient to infer a causal relationship between prenatal and postnatal exposure to secondhand smoke and childhood lymphomas.

6. The evidence is suggestive but not sufficient to infer a causal relationship between prenatal and postnatal exposure to secondhand smoke and childhood brain tumors.
7. The evidence is inadequate to infer the presence or absence of a causal relationship between prenatal and postnatal exposure to secondhand smoke and other childhood cancer types.

Implications

Childhood cancers are diverse in their characteristics and etiology. Although the evidence is inadequate for some sources and periods of exposure, there is some evidence indicative of associations of childhood cancer risk with secondhand smoke exposure. Further research is needed to provide a better understanding of the potential causal relationships between types of exposures to secondhand smoke and childhood cancer risks.

CONCLUSIONS

The following conclusions are supported by text in the full report that may not be included in this excerpt. The full report can be accessed at http://www.surgeongeneral.gov/library/second handsmoke/report/.

Fertility

1. The evidence is inadequate to infer the presence or absence of a causal relationship between maternal exposure to secondhand smoke and female fertility or fecundability. No data were found on paternal exposure to secondhand smoke and male fertility or fecundability.

Pregnancy (Spontaneous Abortion and Perinatal Death)

2. The evidence is inadequate to infer the presence or absence of a causal relationship between maternal exposure to secondhand smoke during pregnancy and spontaneous abortion.

Infant Deaths

3. The evidence is inadequate to infer the presence or absence of a causal relationship between exposure to secondhand smoke and neonatal mortality.

Sudden Infant Death Syndrome

4. The evidence is sufficient to infer a causal relationship between exposure to secondhand smoke and sudden infant death syndrome.

Preterm Delivery

5. The evidence is suggestive but not sufficient to infer a causal relationship between maternal exposure to secondhand smoke during pregnancy and preterm delivery.

Low Birth Weight

6. The evidence is sufficient to infer a causal relationship between maternal exposure to secondhand smoke during pregnancy and a small reduction in birth weight.

Congenital Malformations

7. The evidence is inadequate to infer the presence or absence of a causal relationship between exposure to secondhand smoke and congenital malformations.

Cognitive Development

8. The evidence is inadequate to infer the presence or absence of a causal relationship between exposure to secondhand smoke and cognitive functioning among children.

Behavioral Development

9. The evidence is inadequate to infer the presence or absence of a causal relationship between exposure to secondhand smoke and behavioral problems among children.

Height/Growth

10. The evidence is inadequate to infer the presence or absence of a causal relationship between exposure to secondhand smoke and children's height/growth.

Childhood Cancer

11. The evidence is suggestive but not sufficient to infer a causal relationship between prenatal and postnatal exposure to secondhand smoke and childhood cancer.
12. The evidence is inadequate to infer the presence or absence of a causal relationship between maternal exposure to secondhand smoke during pregnancy and childhood cancer.
13. The evidence is inadequate to infer the presence or absence of a causal relationship between exposure to secondhand smoke during infancy and childhood cancer.
14. The evidence is suggestive but not sufficient to infer a causal relationship between prenatal and postnatal exposure to secondhand smoke and childhood leukemias.
15. The evidence is suggestive but not sufficient to infer a causal relationship between prenatal and postnatal exposure to secondhand smoke and childhood lymphomas.
16. The evidence is suggestive but not sufficient to infer a causal relationship between prenatal and postnatal exposure to secondhand smoke and childhood brain tumors.
17. The evidence is inadequate to infer the presence or absence of a causal relationship between prenatal and postnatal exposure to secondhand smoke and other childhood cancer types.

OVERALL IMPLICATIONS

Because infant mortality for the United States is quite high compared with other industrialized coun tries, identifying strategies to reduce the number of infant deaths should receive high priority. The epide miologic evidence for the association of secondhand smoke exposure and an increased risk of SIDS indi cates that eliminating secondhand smoke exposures among newborns and young infants should be part of an overall strategy to reduce the high infant mortality rate in the United States.

The available evidence for five reproductive and childhood outcomes—childhood cancer, cognitive development, behaviors, LBW, and spontaneous abor tion—calls for further research with improved meth odologies. The methodologic challenges and issues that were discussed in relation to exposure assess ment and reproductive outcomes might act as a guide for future research on these topics. There is a need for studies that examine exposure to secondhand smoke and childhood cancers to further evaluate the risks for specific cancer types. The evidence reviewed in this chapter points to germ-cell mutations among fathers who smoke as a possible pathway. Additional stud ies may be warranted that focus on childhood cancer and active paternal smoking, with improved controls for maternal secondhand smoke exposure and active smoking during pregnancy and the exposure of infants to secondhand smoke. For secondhand smoke and spontaneous abortions, studies using samples with adequate statistical power are needed. For all outcomes, investigations should include biochemical measures of exposures, and these measures should be used to determine the presence of dose-response rela tionships—determining dose-response relationships will greatly facilitate the assessment of causality.

REFERENCES

Ahlborg G Jr, Bodin L. Tobacco smoke exposure and pregnancy outcome among working women: a pro spective study at prenatal care centers in Orebro County, Sweden. *American Journal of Epidemiology.* 1991;133(4):338–47.

American Academy of Pediatrics Task Force on Sud den Infant Death Syndrome. The changing concept of sudden infant death syndrome: diagnostic cod ing shifts, controversies regarding sleeping envi ronment, and new variables to consider reducing risk. *Pediatrics.* 2005;116(5):1245–55.

Anderson HR, Cook DG. Passive smoking and sud den infant death syndrome: review of the epidemi ological evidence. *Thorax.* 1997;52(11):1003–9.

Anderson KN, Anderson LE, Glanze WD, editors. *Mosby's Medical, Nursing, and Allied Health Dictionary.* 5th ed. St. Louis: Mosby-Year Book, 1998.

Andres RL, Day MC. Perinatal complications asso ciated with maternal tobacco use. *Seminars in Neonatology.* 2000;5(3):231–41.

Andresen BD, Ng KJ, Iams JD, Bianchine JR. Cotinine in amniotic fluids from passive smokers [letter]. *Lancet.* 1982;1(8275):791–2.

Augood C, Duckitt K, Templeton AA. Smoking and female infertility: a systematic review and meta analysis. *Human Reproduction.* 1998;13(6):1532–9.

Baghurst PA, Tong SL, Woodward A, McMichael AJ. Effects of maternal smoking upon neuropsycholog ical development in early childhood: importance of taking account of social and environmental factors. *Paediatric and Perinatal Epidemiology.* 1992;6(4):403–15.

Baird DD, Wilcox AJ. Cigarette smoking associated with delayed conception. *Journal of the American Medical Association.* 1985;253(20):2979–83.

Bolumar F, Olsen J, Boldsen J. Smoking reduces fecun dity: a European multicenter study on infertility and subfecundity. *American Journal of Epidemiology.* 1996;143(6):578–87.

Bottoms SF, Kuhnert BR, Kuhnert PM, Reese AL. Maternal passive smoking and fetal serum thio cyanate levels. *American Journal of Obstetrics and Gynecology.* 1982;144(7):787–91.

Bruner JP, Forouzan I. Smoking and buccally adminis tered nicotine: acute effect on uterine and umbilical artery Doppler flow velocity waveforms. *Journal of Reproductive Medicine.* 1991;36(6):435–40.

Bunin GR, Buckley JD, Boesel CP, Rorke LB, Mead ows AT. Risk factors for astrocytic glioma and primitive neuroectodermal tumor of the brain in young children: a report from the Children's Can cer Group. *Cancer Epidemiology, Biomarkers and Prevention.* 1994;3(3):197–204.

California Environmental Protection Agency. *Proposed Identification of Environmental Tobacco Smoke as a Toxic Air Contaminant. Part B: Health Effects.* Sacra mento (CA): California Environmental Protection Agency, Office of Environmental Health Hazard Assessment, 2005.

Cameron P, Kostin JS, Zaks JM, Wolfe JH, Tighe G, Oselett B, Stocker R, Winton J. The health of smok ers' and nonsmokers' children. *Journal of Allergy.* 1969;43(6):336–41.

Chamberlain R. Birthweight and length of gestation. In: Chamberlain R, Chamberlain G, Howlett B, Claireaux A, editors. *British Births. 1970: A*

Survey Under the Joint Auspices of the National Birthday Trust Fund and the Royal College of Obstetricians and Gynaecologists, Volume 1: The First Week of Life. London: William Heinemann Medical Books, 1975:48–88.

Chung PH, Yeko TR, Mayer JC, Clark B, Welden SW, Maroulis GB. Gamete intrafallopian transfer: does smoking play a role? *Journal of Reproductive Medicine.* 1997;42(2):65–70.

Coghlin J, Gann PH, Hammond SK, Skipper PL, Taghizadeh K, Paul M, Tannenbaum SR. 4-Amino biphenyl hemoglobin adducts in fetuses exposed to the tobacco smoke carcinogen in utero. *Journal of the National Cancer Institute.* 1991;83(4):274–80.

Çolak Ö, Alatas Ö, Aydo˘gdu S, Uslu S. The effect of smoking on bone metabolism: maternal and cord blood bone marker levels. *Clinical Biochemistry.* 2002;35(3):247–50.

Coleman S, Piotrow PT, Rinehart W. Tobacco—haz ards to health and human reproduction. *Population Reports Series L, Issues in World Health* 1979;(1): L1–L37.

Colley JRT. Respiratory symptoms in children and parental smoking and phlegm production. *British Medical Journal.* 1974;2(912):201–4.

Colley JR, Holland WW, Corkhill RT. Influence of passive smoking and parental phlegm on pneu monia and bronchitis in early childhood. *Lancet.* 1974;2(7888):1031–4.

Crawford FG, Mayer J, Santella RM, Cooper TB, Ott- man R, Tsai WY, Simon-Cereijido G, Wang M, Tang D, Perera FP. Biomarkers of environmental tobacco smoke in preschool children and their mothers. *Journal of the National Cancer Institute.* 1994;86(18):1398–402.

Daling J, Weiss N, Spadoni L, Moore DE, Voigt L. Cigarette smoking and primary tubal infertility. In: Rosenberg MJ, editor. *Smoking and Reproductive Health.* Littleton (MA): PSG Publishing Company, 1987:40–6.

de Mouzon J, Spira A, Schwartz D. A prospec tive study of the relation between smoking and fertility. *International Journal of Epidemiology.* 1988;17(2):378–84.

Dempsey D, Jacob P III, Benowitz NL. Nicotine metab olism and elimination kinetics in newborns. *Clinical Pharmacology and Therapeutics.* 2000;67(5):458–65.

Dollberg S, Fainaru O, Mimouni FB, Shenhav M, Les- sing JB, Kupferminc M. Effect of passive smoking in pregnancy on neonatal nucleated red blood cells. *Pediatrics.* 2000;106(3):E34.

Dunphy BC, Barratt CL, von Tongelen BP, Cooke ID. Male cigarette smoking and fecundity in couples attending an infertility clinic. *Andrologia.* 1991;23(3):223–5.

Dwyer T, Ponsonby AL, Couper D. Tobacco smoke exposure at one month of age and subsequent risk of SIDS—a prospective study. *American Journal of Epidemiology.* 1999;149(7):593–602.

Elenbogen A, Lipitz S, Mashiach S, Dor J, Levran D, Ben-Rafael Z. The effect of smoking on the outcome of in-vitro fertilization—embryo transfer. *Human Reproduction.* 1991;6(2):242–4.

Emmons KM, Abrams DB, Marshall R, Marcus BH, Kane M, Novotny TE, Etzel RA. An evaluation of the relationship between self-report and biochemi cal measures of environmental tobacco smoke exposure. *Preventive Medicine.* 1994;23(1):35–9.

Ernst M, Moolchan ET, Robinson ML. Behavioral and neural consequences of prenatal exposure to nico tine. *Journal of the American Academy of Child and Adolescent Psychiatry.* 2001;40(6):630–41.

Eskenazi B, Gold EB, Lasley BL, Samuels SJ, Hammond SK, Wight S, O'Neill Rasor M, Hines CJ, Schenker MB. Prospective monitoring of early fetal loss and clinical spontaneous abortion among female semi conductor workers. *American Journal of Industrial Medicine.* 1995;28(6):833–46.

Everson RB, Randerath E, Santella RM, Avitts TA, Weinstein IB, Randerath K. Quantitative associa tions between DNA damage in human placenta and maternal smoking and birth weight. *Journal of the National Cancer Institute.* 1988;80(8):567–76.

Everson RB, Randerath E, Santella RM, Cefalo RC, Avitts TA, Randerath K. Detection of smoking-related covalent DNA adducts in human placenta. *Science.* 1986;231(4733):54–7.

Finette BA, O'Neill JP, Vacek PM, Albertini RJ. Gene mutations with characteristic deletions in cord blood T lymphocytes associated with passive maternal exposure to tobacco smoke. *Nature Medicine* .1998;4(10):1144–51.

Gibson E, Dembofsky CA, Rubin S, Greenspan JS. Infant sleep position practices 2 years into the "Back to Sleep" campaign. *Clinical Pediatrics.* 2000;39(5):285–9.

Goldman LR. Children—unique and vulnerable: envi ronmental risks facing children and recommenda tions for response. *Environmental Health Perspectives.* 1995;103(Suppl 6):13–8.

Gospe SM Jr, Zhou SS, Pinkerton KE. Effects of environmental tobacco smoke exposure in utero and/or postnatally on brain development. *Pediatric Research.* 1996;39(3):494–8.

Greenberg RA, Haley NJ, Etzel RA, Loda FA. Measuring the exposure of infants to tobacco smoke: nicotine and cotinine in urine and saliva. *New England Journal of Medicine.* 1984;310(17):1075–8.

Gruslin A, Perkins SL, Manchanda R, Fleming N, Clinch JJ. Maternal smoking and fetal erythropoietin levels. *Obstetrics and Gynecology.* 2000;95(4):561–4.

Hammond SK. Exposure of U.S. workers to environmental tobacco smoke. *Environmental Health Perspectives.* 1999;107(Suppl 2):329–40.

Hansen C, Sorensen LD, Asmussen I, Autrup H. Transplacental exposure to tobacco smoke in human-adduct formation in placenta and umbilical cord blood vessels. *Teratogenesis, Carcinogenesis, and Mutagenesis.* 1992;12(2):51–60.

Harger JH, Hsing AW, Tuomala RE, Gibbs RS, Mead PB, Eschenbach DA, Knox GE, Polk BF. Risk factors for preterm premature rupture of fetal membranes: a multicenter case-control study. *American Journal of Obstetrics and Gynecology.* 1990;163(1 Pt 1):130–7.

Hauth JC, Hauth J, Drawbaugh RB, Gilstrap LC 3rd, Pierson WP. Passive smoking and thiocyanate concentrations in pregnant women and newborns. *Obstetrics and Gynecology.* 1984;63(4):519–22.

Howe GR, Burch JD, Chiarelli AM, Risch HA, Choi BC. An exploratory case-control study of brain tumors in children. *Cancer Research.* 1989;49(15):4349–52.

Hughes EG, Brennan BG. Does cigarette smoking impair natural or assisted fecundity? *Fertility and Sterility.* 1996;66(5):679–89.

Hughes EG, YoungLai EV, Ward SM. Cigarette smoking and outcomes of in-vitro fertilization and embryo transfer: a prospective cohort study. *Human Reproduction.* 1992;7(3):358–61.

Hull MG, North K, Taylor H, Farrow A, Ford WC. Delayed conception and active and passive smoking. *Fertility and Sterility.* 2000;74(4):725–33.

Hwang SJ, Beaty TH, Panny SR, Street NA, Joseph JM, Gordon S, McIntosh I, Francomano CA. Association study of transforming growth factor alpha (TGF alpha) TaqI polymorphism and oral clefts: indication of gene-environment interaction in a population-based sample of infants with birth defects. *American Journal of Epidemiology.* 1995;141(7):629–36.

Jaakkola JJ, Jaakkola N, Zahlsen K. Fetal growth and length of gestation in relation to prenatal exposure to environmental tobacco smoke assessed by hair nicotine concentration. *Environmental Health Perspectives.* 2001;109(6):557–61.

Jazayeri A, Tsibris JC, Spellacy WN. Umbilical cord plasma erythropoietin levels in pregnancies com plicated by maternal smoking. *American Journal of Obstetrics and Gynecology.* 1998;178(3):433–5.

Joad JP. Smoking and pediatric respiratory health. *Clinics in Chest Medicine.* 2000;21(1):37–46, vii–viii.

Kaufman FL, Kharrazi M, Delorenze GN, Eskenazi B, Bernert JT. Estimation of environmental tobacco smoke exposure during pregnancy using a single question on household smokers versus serum coti nine. *Journal of Exposure Analysis and Environmental Epidemiology.* 2002;12(4):286–95.

Klonoff-Cohen HS, Edelstein SL, Lefkowitz ES, Srinivasan IP, Kaegi D, Chang JC, Wiley KJ. The effect of passive smoking and tobacco exposure through breast milk on sudden infant death syn drome. *Journal of the American Medical Association.* 1995;273(10):795–8.

Koo LC, Ho JH, Rylander R. Life-history correlates of environmental tobacco smoke: a study on non smoking Hong Kong Chinese wives with smoking versus nonsmoking husbands. *Social Science and Medicine.* 1988;26(7):751–60.

Kuijten RR, Bunin GR, Nass CC, Meadows AT. Ges tational and familial risk factors for childhood astrocytoma: results of a case-control study. *Cancer. Research* 1990;50(9):2608–12.

Lambers DS, Clark KE. The maternal and fetal physi ologic effects of nicotine. *Seminars in Perinatology.* 1996;20(2):115–26.

Lammer EJ, Shaw GM, Iovannisci DM, Van Waes J, Finnell RH. Maternal smoking and the risk of oro facial clefts: susceptibility with *NAT1* and *NAT2* polymorphisms. *Epidemiology.* 2004;15(2):150–6.

Laurent SL, Thompson SJ, Addy C, Garrison CZ, Moore EE. An epidemiologic study of smoking and primary infertility in women. *Fertility and Sterility.* 1992;57(3):565–72.

Li CQ, Windsor RA, Perkins L, Goldenberg RL, Lowe JB. The impact on infant birth weight and gesta tional age of cotinine-validated smoking reduction during pregnancy. *Journal of the American Medical Association.* 1993;269(12):1519–24.

Lindbohm ML, Sallmen M, Taskinen H. Effects of exposure to environmental tobacco smoke on reproductive health. *Scandinavian Journal of Work, Environment and Health.* 2002;28(Suppl 2):84–96.

Little J, Cardy A, Arslan MT, Gilmour M, Mossey PA. Smoking and orofacial clefts: a United Kingdom- based case-control study. *The Cleft Palate-Craniofacial Journal.* 2004a;41(4):381–6.

Little J, Cardy A, Munger RG. Tobacco smoking and oral clefts: a meta-analysis. *Bulletin of the World Health Organization.* 2004b;82(3):213–8.

Longo FJ, Anderson E. The effects of nicotine on fertilization in the sea urchin, *Arbacia punctulata. Journal of Cell Biology.* 1970;46(2):308–25.

Machaalani R, Waters KA, Tinworth KD. Effects of postnatal nicotine exposure on apoptotic markers in the developing piglet brain. *Neuroscience.* 2005;132(2):325–33.

Maier RF, Bohme K, Dudenhausen JW, Obladen M. Cord blood erythropoietin in relation to different markers of fetal hypoxia. *Obstetrics and Gynecology.* 1993;81(4):575–80.

Mainous AG 3rd, Hueston WJ. The effect of smoking cessation during pregnancy on preterm delivery and low birthweight. *Journal of Family Practice.* 1994;38(3):262–6.

Malloy MH. Trends in postneonatal aspiration deaths and reclassification of sudden infant death syndrome: impact of the "Back to Sleep" program. *Pediatrics.* 2002;109(4):661–5.

Malloy MH, Freeman DH. Age at death, season, and day of death as indicators of the effect of the Back to Sleep program on sudden infant death syndrome in the United States, 1992–1999. *Archives of Pediatrics and Adolescent Medicine.* 2004;158(4):359–65.

Manchester DK, Jacoby EH. Sensitivity of human placental monooxygenase activity to maternal smoking. *Clinical Pharmacology and Therapeutics.* 1981;30(5):687–92.

Marcus BH, Emmons KM, Abrams DB, Marshall RJ, Kane M, Novotny TE, Etzel RA. Restrictive work place smoking policies: impact on nonsmokers' tobacco exposure. *Journal of Public Health Policy.* 1992;13(1):42–51.

Martin JA, Hamilton BE, Sutton PD, Ventura SJ, Menacker F, Munson ML. Births: final data for 2003. *National Vital Statistics Reports.* 2005;54(2):1–116.

Mathews TJ, Menacker F, MacDorman MF. Infant mortality statistics from the 2002 period: linked birth/infant death data set. *National Vital Statistics Reports.* 2004;53(10):1–32.

Mattison DR. The effects of smoking on fertility from gametogenesis to implantation. *Environmental Research.* 1982;28(2):410–33.

Mattison DR, Plowchalk DR, Meadows MJ, Miller MM, Malek A, London S. The effect of smoking on oogenesis, fertilization, and implantation. *Seminars in Reproductive Endocrinology.* 1989;7(4):291–304.

Mattison DR, Thomford PJ. The effect of smoking on reproductive ability and reproductive lifespan. In: Rosenberg MJ, editor. *Smoking and*

Reproductive Health. Littleton (MA): PSG Publishing Company, 1987:47–54.

McCann MF, Irwin DE, Walton LA, Hulka BS, Mor ton JL, Axelrad CM. Nicotine and cotinine in the cervical mucus of smokers, passive smokers, and nonsmokers. *Cancer Epidemiology, Biomarkers and Prevention.* 1992;1(2):125–9.

Meyer KA, Williams P, Hernandez-Diaz S, Cnat tingius S. Smoking and the risk of oral clefts: exploring the impact of study designs. *Epidemiology.* 2004;15(6):671–8.

Misra DP, Nguyen RH. Environmental tobacco smoke and low birth weight: a hazard in the workplace? *Environmental Health Perspectives.* 1999;107(Suppl 6):897–904.

Mohr U, Reznik-Schuller H, Reznik G, Hilfrich J. Transplacental effects of diethylnitrosamine in Syr ian hamsters as related to different days of admin istration during pregnancy. *Journal of the National Cancer Institute.* 1975;55(3):681–3.

Naeye RL. Abruptio placentae and placenta previa: frequency, perinatal mortality, and cigarette smok ing. *Obstetrics and Gynecology.* 1980;55(6):701–4.

Napalkov NP. Some general considerations on the problem of transplacental carcinogenesis. In: Tom atis L, Mohr U, Davis W, editors. *Transplacental Carcinogenesis.* IARC Scientific Publications No. 4. Lyon (France): International Agency for Research on Cancer, 1973:1–13.

Napalkov NP, Rice JM, Tomatis L, Yamasaki H, edi tors. *Perinatal and Multigeneration Carcinogenesis.* IARC Scientific Publications No. 96. Lyon (France): International Agency for Research on Cancer, 1989.

National Cancer Institute. *Health Effects of Exposure to Environmental Tobacco Smoke: The Report of the California Environmental Protection Agency.* Smoking and Tobacco Control Monograph No. 10. Bethesda (MD): U.S. Department of Health and Human Services, National Institutes of Health, National Cancer Institute, 1999. NIH Pub. No. 99-4645.

Nebert DW, Winker J, Gelboin HV. Aryl hydrocar bon hydroxylase activity in human placenta from cigarette smoking and nonsmoking women. *Cancer Research.* 1969;29(10):1763–9.

Neri A, Marcus SL. Effect of nicotine on the motil ity of the oviducts in the rhesus monkey: a pre liminary report. *Journal of Reproduction and Fertility.* 1972;31(1):91–7.

Nicolov IG, Chernozemsky IN. Tumors and hyper plastic lesions in Syrian hamsters following trans placental and neonatal treatment with cigarette smoke condensate. *Journal of Cancer Research and Clinical Oncology.* 1979;94(3):249–56.

Ownby DR, Johnson CC, Peterson EL. Passive ciga rette smoke exposure in infants: importance of nonparental sources. *Archives of Pediatrics and Adolescent Medicine.* 2000;154(12):1237–41.

Pacifici R, Altieri I, Gandini L, Lenzi A, Passa AR, Pichini S, Rosa M, Zuccaro P, Dondero F. Envi ronmental tobacco smoke: nicotine and cotinine concentration in semen. *Environmental Research.* 1995;68(1):69–72.

Pattinson HA, Taylor PJ, Pattinson MH. The effect of cigarette smoking on ovarian function and early pregnancy outcome of in vitro fertilization treat ment. *Fertility and Sterility.* 1991;55(4):780–3.

Pattishall EN, Strope GL, Etzel RA, Helms RW, Haley NJ, Denny FW. Serum cotinine as a measure of tobacco smoke exposure in children. *American Journal of Diseases of Children.* 1985;139(11):1101–4.

Pirkle JL, Flegal KM, Bernert JT, Brody DJ, Etzel RA, Maurer KR. Exposure of the US population to environmental tobacco smoke: the Third National Health and Nutrition Examination Survey, 1988 to 1991. *Journal of the American Medical Association.* 1996;275(16):1233–40.

Ponsonby AL, Dwyer T, Cochrane J. Population trends in sudden infant death syndrome. *Seminars in Perinatology.* 2002;26(4):296–305.

Preston-Martin S, Yu MC, Benton B, Henderson BE. *N*-Nitroso compounds and childhood brain tumors: a case-control study. *Cancer Research.* 1982;42(12):5240–5.

Prokopczyk B, Cox JE, Hoffmann D, Waggoner SE. Identification of tobacco-specific carcinogen in the cervical mucus of smokers and nonsmokers. *Journal of the National Cancer Institute.* 1997;89(12):868–73.

Rajini P, Last JA, Pinkerton KE, Hendrickx AG, Wits- chi H. Decreased fetal weights in rats exposed to sidestream cigarette smoke. *Fundamental and Applied Toxicology.* 1994;22(3):400–4.

Rebagliato M, Bolumar F, Florey C du V. Assessment of exposure to environmental tobacco smoke in nonsmoking pregnant women in different envi ronments of daily living. *American Journal of Epidemiology.* 1995;142(5):525–30.

Rice JM. Perinatal period and pregnancy: intervals of high risk for chemical carcinogens. *Environmental Health Perspectives.* 1979;29:23–7.

Rice JM, Rehm S, Donovan PJ, Perantoni AO. Compar ative transplacental carcinogenesis by directly act ing and metabolism-dependent alkylating agents in rodents and nonhuman primates. In: Napalkov NP, Rice JM, Tomatis L,

Yamasaki H, editors. *Perinatal and Multigeneration Carcinogenesis.* IARC Scientific Publications No. 96. Lyon (France): International Agency for Research on Cancer, 1989:17–34.

Rosenberg MJ. Does smoking affect sperm? In: Rosenberg MJ, editor. *Smoking and Reproductive Health.* Littleton (MA): PSG Publishing Company, 1987:54–62.

Rosevear SK, Holt DW, Lee TD, Ford WC, Wardle PG, Hull MG. Smoking and decreased fertilisation rates in vitro. *Lancet.* 1992;340(8829):1195–6.

Rowlands DJ, McDermott A, Hull MG. Smoking and decreased fertilisation rates in vitro [letter]. *Lancet.* 1992;340(8832):1409–10.

Ruckebusch Y. Relationship between the electrical activity of the oviduct and the uterus of the rabbit in vivo. *Journal of Reproduction and Fertility.* 1975;45(1):73–82.

Sadler TW. *Langman's Medical Embryology.* 6th ed. Baltimore: Williams and Wilkins, 1990.

Sasson IM, Haley NJ, Hoffman D, Wynder EL, Hellberg D, Nilsson S. Cigarette smoking and neoplasia of the uterine cervix: smoke constituents in cervical mucus [letter]. *New England Journal of Medicine.* 1985;312(5):315–6.

Schuller HM, editor. *Comparative Perinatal Carcinogenesis.* Boca Raton (FL): CRC Press, 1984.

Seidman DS, Mashiach S. Involuntary smoking and pregnancy. *European Journal of Obstetrics, Gynecology, and Reproductive Biology.* 1991;41(2):105–16.

Shaw GM, Wasserman CR, Lammer EJ, O'Malley CD, Murray JC, Basart AM, Tolarova MM. Orofacial clefts, parental cigarette smoking, and transforming growth factor-alpha gene variants. *American Journal of Human Genetics.* 1996;58(3):551–61.

Slotkin TA. Fetal nicotine or cocaine exposure: which one is worse? *Journal of Pharmacology and Experimental Therapy.* 1998;285(3):931–45.

Slotkin TA, Pinkerton KE, Garofolo MC, Auman JT, McCook EC, Seidler FJ. Perinatal exposure to environmental tobacco smoke induces adenyl cyclase and alters receptor-mediated cell signaling in brain and heart of neonatal rats. *Brain Research.* 2001;898(1):73–81.

Slotkin TA, Pinkerton KE, Seidler FJ. Perinatal environmental tobacco smoke exposure in rhesus monkeys: critical periods and regional selectivity for effects on brain cell development and lipid peroxidation. *Environmental Health Perspectives.* 2006;114(1):34–9.

Smith CJ, Livingston SD, Doolittle DJ. An international literature survey of "IARC Group I carcinogens" reported in mainstream cigarette smoke. *Food and Chemical Toxicology.* 1997;35(10–11):1107–30.

Smith CJ, Perfetti TA, Mullens MA, Rodgman A, Doo little DJ. "IARC group 2B Carcinogens" reported in cigarette mainstream smoke. *Food and Chemical Toxicology.* 2000a;38(9):825–48.

Smith CJ, Perfetti TA, Rumple MA, Rodgman A, Doo little DJ. "IARC group 2A Carcinogens" reported in cigarette mainstream smoke. *Food and Chemical Toxicology.* 2000b;38(4):371–83.

Smith N, Austen J, Rolles CJ. Tertiary smoking by the fetus [letter]. *Lancet.* 1982;1(8283):1252–3.

Stavrou D, Dahme E, Haenichen T. Transplacental carcinogenesis in the rabbit. In: Schuller HM, edi tor. *Comparative Perinatal Carcinogenesis.* Boca Raton (FL): CRC Press, 1984:23–43.

Stick SM, Burton PR, Gurrin L, Sly PD, LeSouef PH. Effects of maternal smoking during pregnancy and a family history of asthma on respiratory function in newborn infants. *Lancet.* 1996;348(9034):1060–4.

Stillman RJ, Rosenberg MJ, Sachs BP. Smoking and reproduction. *Fertility and Sterility.* 1986;46(4):545–66.

Suonio S, Saarikoski S, Kauhanen O, Metsapelto A, Terho J, Vohlonen I. Smoking does affect fecundity. *European Journal of Obstetrics, Gynecology, and Reproductive Biology* 1990;34(1–2):89–95.

Tokuhata GK. Smoking in relation to infertility and fetal loss. *Archives of Environmental Health.* 1968;17(3):353–9.

Trapp M, Kemeter P, Feichtinger W. Smoking and in-vitro fertilization. *Human Reproduction* 1986;1(6):357–8.

Underwood PB, Kesler KF, O'Lane JJ, Callagan DA. Parental smoking empirically related to pregnancy outcome. *Obstetrics and Gynecology.* 1967;29(1):1–8.

United Kingdom Department of Health. *Report of the Scientific Committee on Tobacco and Health.* Norwich (United Kingdom): The Stationery Office, 1998. (See also <http://www.archive.official-documents.co.uk/document/doh/tobacco/contents.htm>; accessed: June 26, 2003.)

U.S. Department of Health and Human Services. *The Health Consequences of Smoking for Women. A Report of the Surgeon General.* Washington: U.S. Department of Health and Human Services, Public Health Service, Office of the Assistant Secretary for Health, Office on Smoking and Health, 1980.

U.S. Department of Health and Human Services. *The Health Consequences of Involuntary Smoking. A Report of the Surgeon General.* Rockville (MD): U.S. Department of Health and Human Services, Public Health Service, Centers for

Disease Control, Center for Health Promotion and Education, Office on Smoking and Health, 1986. DHHS Publication No. (CDC) 87-8398.

U.S. Department of Health and Human Services. *The Health Benefits of Smoking Cessation. A Report of the Surgeon General.* Atlanta: U.S. Department of Health and Human Services, Public Health Service, Centers for Disease Control, National Center for Chronic Disease Prevention and Health Promotion, Office on Smoking and Health, 1990. DHHS Publi cation No. (CDC) 90-8416.

U.S. Department of Health and Human Services. *Women and Smoking. A Report of the Surgeon General.* Rockville (MD): U.S. Department of Health and Human Services, Public Health Service, Office of the Surgeon General, 2001.

U.S. Department of Health and Human Services. *The Health Consequences of Smoking: A Report of the Surgeon General.* Atlanta: U.S. Department of Health and Human Services, Centers for Disease Control and Prevention, National Center for Chronic Dis ease Prevention and Health Promotion, Office on Smoking and Health, 2004.

U.S. Department of Health and Human Services. *The Health Consequences of Involuntary Exposure to Tobacco Smoke: A Report of the Surgeon General.* Atlanta: U.S. Department of Health and Human Services, Centers for Disease Control and Prevention, National Center for Chronic Disease Prevention and Health Promotion, Office on Smoking and Health, 2006.

U.S. Department of Health, Education, and Welfare. *Smoking and Health: Report of the Advisory Committee to the Surgeon General of the Public Health Service.* Washington: U.S. Department of Health, Educa tion, and Welfare, Public Health Service, Center for Disease Control, 1964. PHS Publication No. 1103.

U.S. Department of Health, Education, and Welfare. *The Health Consequences of Smoking. A Report of the Surgeon General, 1974.* Washington: U.S. Depart ment of Health, Education, and Welfare, Public Health Service, Center for Disease Control, 1974. DHEW Publication No. (CDC) 74-8704.

U.S. Department of Health, Education, and Welfare. *Smoking and Health. A Report of the Surgeon General.* Washington: U.S. Department of Health, Education, and Welfare, Public Health Service, Office of the Assistant Secretary for Health, Office of Smoking and Health, 1979a. DHEW Publication No. (PHS) 79-50066.

U.S. Department of Health, Education, and Welfare. *The Health Consequences of Smoking. A Report of the Surgeon General, 1977–1978.* Rockville (MD): U.S. Department of Health and Human Services, Public Health Service, Office

of the Assistant Secretary for Health, Office on Smoking and Health, 1979b. DHEW Publication No. (CDC) 79-50065.
University of Toronto. *Protection From Second-Hand Tobacco Smoke in Ontario: A Review of the Evidence Regarding Best Practices.* Toronto: University of Toronto, Ontario Tobacco Research Unit, 2001.
van den Berg BJ, Oechsli FW. Prematurity. In: Bracken MB, editor. *Perinatal Epidemiology.* New York: Oxford University Press, 1984:69–85.
van Rooij IALM, Groenen PMW, van Drongelen M, te Morsche RHM, Peters WHM, Steegers-Theunissen RPM. Orofacial clefts and spina bifida: N-acetyl transferase phenotype, maternal smoking, and medication use. *Teratology.* 2002;66(5):260–6.
van Rooij IALM, Wegerif MJM, Roelofs HMJ, Peters WHM, Kuijpers-Jagtman A-M, Zielhuis GA, Merkus HMWM, Steegers-Theunissen RPM. Smoking, genetic polymorphisms in biotransfor mation enzymes, and nonsyndromic oral clefting: a gene-environment interaction. *Epidemiology.* 2001;12(5):502–7.
Van Voorhis BJ, Syrop CH, Hammitt DG, Dunn MS, Snyder GD. Effects of smoking on ovulation induc tion for assisted reproductive techniques. *Fertility and Sterility.* 1992;58(5):981–5.
Vessey MP. Epidemiological studies of the effects of diethylstilbestrol. In: Napalkov NP, Rice JM, Tom atis L, Yamasaki H, editors. *Perinatal and Multigeneration Carcinogenesis.* IARC Scientific Publications No. 96. Lyon (France): International Agency for Research on Cancer, 1989:335–48.
Vine MF, Margolin BH, Morrison HI, Hulka BS. Ciga rette smoking and sperm density: a meta-analysis. *Fertility and Sterility.* 1994;61(1):35–43.
Weiss T, Eckert A. Cotinine levels in follicular fluid and serum of IVF patients: effect on granulosaluteal cell function in vitro. *Human Reproduction.* 1989;4(5):482–5.
Werler MM. Teratogen update: smoking and reproductive outcomes. *Teratology.* 1997;55(6):382–8.
Wilcox AJ. Birth weight and perinatal mortality: the effect of maternal smoking. *American Journal of Epidemiology.* 1993;137(10):1098–104.
Wilcox AJ, Weinberg CR, O'Connor JF, Baird DD, Schlatterer JP, Canfield RE, Armstrong EG, Nisula BC. Incidence of early loss of pregnancy. *New England Journal of Medicine.* 1988;319(4):189–94.
Williams MA, Mittendorf R, Stubblefield PG, Lieber man E, Schoenbaum SC, Monson RR. Cigarettes, coffee, and preterm premature rupture of the membranes. *American Journal of Epidemiology.* 1992;135(8):895–903.

Windham GC, Eaton A, Hopkins B. Evidence for an association between environmental tobacco smoke exposure and birthweight: a meta-analysis and new data. *Paediatric and Perinatal Epidemiology.* 1999a;13(1):35–57.

Windham GC, Von Behren J, Waller K, Fenster L. Exposure to environmental and mainstream tobacco smoke and risk of spontaneous abortion. *American Journal of Epidemiology.* 1999b;149(3):243–7.

World Health Organization. *International Consultation on Environmental Tobacco Smoke (ETS) and Child Health: Consultation Report.* Geneva: World Health Organization, Tobacco Free Initiative, 1999. Report No. WHO/NCD/TFI/99.10.

Wyszynski DF, Duffy DL, Beaty TH. Maternal cigarette smoking and oral clefts: a meta-analysis. *Cleft Palate-Craniofacial Journal.* 1997;34(3):206–10.

Yeruchimovich M, Dollberg S, Green DW, Mimouni FB. Nucleated red blood cells in infants of smoking mothers. *Obstetrics and Gynecology.* 1999;93(3):403–6.

Yoshinaga K, Rice C, Krenn J. Effects of nicotine on early pregnancy in the rat. *Biology of Reproduction.* 1979;20(2):294–303.

Zenzes MT, Puy LA, Bielecki R. Immunodetection of benzo[*a*]pyrene adducts in ovarian cells of women exposed to cigarette smoke. *Molecular Human Reproduction.* 1998;4(2):159–65.

Zenzes MT, Reed TE, Wang P, Klein J. Cotinine, a major metabolite of nicotine, is detectable in follicular fluids of passive smokers in in vitro fertilization therapy. *Fertility and Sterility.* 1996;66(4):614–9.

Chapter 4

EXCERPTS FROM CHAPTER 6. RESPIRATORY EFFECTS IN CHILDREN FROM EXPOSURE TO SECONDHAND SMOKE

INTRODUCTION

Adverse effects of parental smoking on the respiratory health of children have been a clinical and public health concern for decades. As early as 1974, two articles published in the journal *Lancet* alerted readers to a possible link between parental smoking and the risk of a lower respiratory illness (LRI) among infants (Colley et al. 1974; Harlap and Davies 1974). Although adverse effects on children from exposure to second hand tobacco smoke had already been suggested (Cameron et al. 1969; Norman-Taylor and Dickinson 1972), the association with early episodes of acute chest illnesses was of immediate and continuing interest because of the suspected long-term consequences for lung growth, chronic respiratory morbidity in childhood, and adult chronic obstructive lung disease (Samet et al. 1983).

Subsequently, many epidemiologic studies have associated parental smoking with respiratory diseases and other adverse health effects throughout childhood. The exposures covered include maternal smoking during pregnancy and afterward, paternal smoking, parental smoking generally, and smoking by others. In 1986, the evidence was sufficient for the U.S. Surgeon General to conclude that the children of parents who smoked had an increased frequency of acute respiratory illnesses and related hospital admissions during infancy (U.S. Department of Health and Human Services [USDHHS] 1986). The 1986 Surgeon General's report also noted that in older children, there was an increased frequency of cough and phlegm and some evidence of an association with middle ear disease. The report also commented on an association between slowed lung growth in children and parental smoking. Several authoritative reviews by various agencies followed the 1986 report (U.S. Environ mental Protection Agency [USEPA] 1992; National Cancer Institute [NCI] 1999). Some researchers have systematically reviewed the literature and, where appropriate, carried out meta-analyses (DiFranza and Lew 1996; Uhari et al. 1996; Li et al. 1999); the most comprehensive systematic review was commissioned by the Department of Health in England (Scientific Committee on Tobacco and Health 1998). Updated ver sions of these reviews were then published as a series of articles in the journal *Thorax* (Cook and Strachan 1997, 1998, 1999; Strachan and Cook 1997, 1998a,b,c; Cook et al. 1998). These papers later served as a foundation for the 1999 World Health Organization (WHO) consultation report on environmental tobacco smoke and child health (WHO 1999). This chapter of the Surgeon General's report presents a major update of those reviews based on literature searches carried out through March 2001. The methodology for these reviews is described later in this chapter (see "Meth ods Used to Review the Evidence"). Selected key references published subsequent to these reviews are included in an appendix of significant additions to the literature at the end of this report.

The section that follows focuses on the biologic basis for respiratory health effects; Chapter 2 (Toxi cology of Secondhand Smoke) in the full report pro vides further background. Separate sections in the full report review the evidence for different adverse effects of secondhand smoke exposure of children: LRIs in infancy and early childhood, middle ear disease and adenotonsillectomy, frequency of respiratory symp toms and prevalent asthma in school-age children, and cohort and case-control studies of the onset of asthma in childhood. There is also a review of the evidence for the effects of parental smoking on several physi ologic measures, lung function, bronchial reactivity, and atopic sensitization. Each section concludes with a summary and an interpretation of the evidence.

The epidemiologic evidence is reviewed in detail in the full report. Therefore, it is not included in this Excerpt. The full report may be accessed at http://www.surgeongeneral.gov/library/secondhandsmoke/report.

MECHANISMS OF HEALTH EFFECTS FROM SECONDHAND TOBACCO SMOKE

This section reviews the biologic impact of secondhand smoke on the respiratory system of the child. Subsequent sections summarize the evidence for adverse health effects on infants and children and describe postulated mechanisms for these effects. Chapter 2 in the full report provides additional gen eral data on these mechanisms.

Introduction

Pregnant women who smoke expose the fetus to tobacco smoke components during a critical win dow of lung development, with consequences that may be persistent. In infancy and early childhood, the contributions of prenatal versus postnatal exposures to secondhand smoke are difficult to separate because women who smoke during pregnancy almost invari ably continue to smoke after their children are born. For children, exposure to secondhand smoke may lead to respiratory illnesses as a result of adverse effects on the immune system and on lung growth and develop ment.

Lung Development and Growth

Active smoking by the mother during pregnancy has causal adverse effects on pregnancy outcomes that are well documented (USDHHS 2001, 2004). Exposure of pregnant women to secondhand tobacco smoke has also been associated with prematurity (Hanke et al. 1999), reduced birth weight (Mainous and Hueston 1994; Misra and Nguyen 1999), and small for gesta tional age outcomes in some studies (Dejin-Karlsson et al. 1998). However, the developmental effects on the respiratory system from maternal smoking dur ing pregnancy extend beyond those that might be expected based on prematurity alone—the airways are particularly affected. Studies have demonstrated that lower measured airflows associated with second hand smoke exposure are not completely explained by the reduction in somatic growth caused by mater nal smoking (Young et al. 2000b). Researchers suspect that fetal growth limitations are mediated in part by the vasoconstrictive effects of nicotine, which may limit uterine blood flow and induce fetal hypoxia (Philipp et al. 1984). Fetal hypoxia, in turn, may lead to slowed fetal growth and may have direct effects on the lung, possibly affecting lung mechanics by suppressing the fetal respiratory rate. Studies have demonstrated a decrease in fetal movement for at least one hour after maternal smoking, which is consistent with fetal hypoxia (Thaler et al. 1980). Smoking dur ing pregnancy may also negatively affect the control of respiration in the fetus (Lewis and Bosque 1995).

Researchers have proposed several mechanisms that explain the effects of maternal smoking during pregnancy on infant lung function. Animal and human studies suggest that morphologic and metabolic alter ations result from in utero exposure to tobacco smoke components that cross the placental barrier (Bassi et al. 1984; Philipp et al. 1984; Collins et al. 1985; Chen et al. 1987). One study with monkeys that involved infusion of nicotine into the mother during pregnancy showed lung hypoplasia and changes in the devel oping alveoli (Sekhon et al. 1999). The investigators postulated that the effect was mediated by the nico tine cholinergic receptors, which showed an increased expansion and binding with nicotine administration. Further research with this model indicated altered collagen in the developing lung (Sekhon et al. 2002). Studies with this and similar models have shown a variety of effects from nicotine on the neonatal lung (Pierce and Nguyen 2002). The programming of fetal growth genes in utero may have a lifelong effect on lung development and disease susceptibility, areas of ongoing research in other diseases. There is now sub stantial research in progress on early life events and future disease risk that follows the general hypothesis proposed by Barker and colleagues (1996).

Exposure to secondhand smoke may also lead to structural changes in the developing lung. In a rat model, Collins and colleagues (1985) found that intra uterine exposure of the pregnant rat to secondhand smoke was associated with pulmonary hypoplasia in the baby rats with decreased lung volumes; in this rat model, exposure reduced the number of sacules but increased their size. Brown and colleagues (1995) assessed respiratory mechanics in 53 healthy infants, and interpreted the pattern of findings to suggest that prenatal tobacco smoke exposure from smoking by the mother may lead to a reduction in airway size and changes in lung properties.

Lung maturation in utero is regulated by the endocrine environment, and the timing of secondhand smoke exposures with regard to lung development may have a lifelong impact on respiratory function. Secondhand smoke components may increase in utero stress responses that then speed lung maturation at the expense of lung growth. Several studies have demonstrated an effect on the fetal endocrine milieu secondary to secondhand smoke exposure (Divers et al. 1981; Catlin et al. 1990; Lieberman et al. 1992). Stud ies have also associated maternal smoking with more advanced lung maturity measured by lectin/sphin gomyelin (L/S) ratios that were out of proportion to fetal size in human infants (Mainous and Hueston 1994). Cotinine levels measured in the amniotic fluid were positively correlated with L/S ratios. Studies also noted an increase in free, conjugated, and total cortisol levels, suggesting a potentially direct or indi rect role for hormonal effects of secondhand smoke on the fetus (Lieberman et al. 1992). Other researchers have demonstrated higher levels of catecholamines in amniotic fluid in pregnant smokers compared with pregnant nonsmokers, further supporting an endo crine mechanism for the effect of secondhand smoke (Divers et al. 1981).

Multiple studies suggest that the effect of secondhand smoke on the development of the respi ratory system begins with in utero exposure (Tager et al. 1995; Stick et al. 1996; Lodrup Carlsen et al. 1997). Stick and colleagues (1996) reported a dose-dependent effect of in utero cigarette smoke exposure in decreas ing tidal flow patterns that were measured during the first three days of life (i.e., before any postnatal exposure). This effect was independent of the effect of smoking on birth weight. Hoo and colleagues (1998) evaluated respiratory function in preterm infants of mothers who did and did not smoke during preg nancy, with the goal of investigating whether the effect of prenatal tobacco smoke exposure is limited to an influence during the last weeks of gestation. The researchers observed that respiratory function was impaired in infants born preterm (an average of seven weeks early), suggesting that the adverse effect of prenatal tobacco smoke exposure is not limited to the last weeks of in utero development. The ratio of time to peak tidal expiratory flow to expiratory time (TPTEF:TE) was lower in infants exposed to sec ondhand smoke in utero compared with unexposed infants (mean 0.369 standard deviation [SD] 0.109 ver sus mean 0.426 SD 0.135, p 0.02). Because TPTEF:TE is associated with airway caliber, these data imply that cigarette smoke exposure in utero may affect airway development. Lower maximal forced expiratory flow at functional residual capacity (VmaxFRC) (Hanrahan et al. 1992) and diminished expiratory flows (Brown et al. 1995) in infants exposed in utero to secondhand smoke provide further support for the contention that infants of mothers who smoke during pregnancy have smaller airways. Increased airway wall thickness and increased smooth muscle, which can both lead to a decreased airway diameter, were found in infants exposed to tobacco smoke in utero who had died of sudden infant death syndrome (SIDS) (Elliot et al. 1999). In animal models of secondhand smoke expo sure, fetuses of rats exposed to mainstream smoke (from active smoking) or to secondhand (sidestream) smoke had reduced lung volume, decreased elastic tissue within the parenchyma, increased density of interstitial tissue, and inadequate development of elastin and collagen (Collins et al. 1985; Vidic 1991). These animal and human data provide clear evidence for an adverse effect of in utero exposure to tobacco smoke on the developing lung. Studies also document structural changes in animal models and in exposed children who have died from SIDS. The physiologic findings suggest altered lung mechanics and reduced airflow consistent with changes in structure.

Immunologic Effects and Inflammation

The development of lung immunophenotype (i.e., the pattern of immunologic response in the lung) is considered to have a key role in determining the risk for asthma, particularly in regard to the T-helper 1 (Th1) pathway (which mediates cellular immunity) and the Th2 pathway (which mediates allergic responses). Secondhand smoke exposure may promote immuno logic development along Th2 pathways, thus contrib uting to the intermediate phenotypes associated with asthma and with a predilection to chronic respiratory disease. Gene-environment interactions that begin in utero and persist during critical periods of develop ment after birth represent the least understood, but potentially the most important, mechanistic route for a lasting influence of secondhand smoke. Although a meta-analysis of epidemiologic evidence suggests that parental smoking before birth (or early childhood secondhand smoke exposure) does not increase the risk for allergic sensitization, other lines of mechanis tic investigation do show a variety of influences from secondhand smoke on immune and inflammatory responses (Strachan and Cook 1998b).

Secondhand smoke effects on T cells may influ ence gene regulation, inflammatory cell function, cytokine production, and immunoglobulin E (IgE) synthesis. These effects are particularly important to consider in regard to immune system ontogeny and for the subsequent development of allergies in childhood. Researchers have demonstrated that mainstream and sidestream smoke condensates selectively suppress the interferon gamma induction of several macrophage functions, including phago cytosis of Ig-opsonized sheep red blood cells, class II major histocompatibility complex expression, and nitric oxide synthesis, which are all representative of effects on immunity (Braun et al. 1998; Edwards et al. 1999). Alterations in antigen presentation may occur not only in the respiratory tract but also in the rest of the body where absorbed toxicants are dis tributed. Macrophages are potent effector cells for immune responsiveness; suppression of their ability to respond to environmental challenges could have lifelong consequences on immune function.

Immune responses may also be increased as a result of secondhand smoke exposure. Animal stud ies demonstrate increases in IgE, eosinophils, and Th2 cytokines (especially interleukin [IL]-4 and IL-10) with exposure to secondhand smoke. These increases may augment the potential for allergic sensitization and the development of an atopy phenotype. In mice sensitized to the ovalbumin (OVA) antigen and exposed to secondhand smoke for six hours per day, five days per week, for six weeks, researchers mea sured increases in total IgE, OVA-specific immuno globulin G1, and eosinophils in the blood (Seymour et al. 1997). These measures indicate an increase in the allergic response to inhaled antigens. On the basis of the results from this mouse model, the investigators concluded that allergen sensitization with the increase in Th2 responses may contribute to the development of allergies in individuals exposed to secondhand smoke (Seymour et al. 1997). Other studies have dem onstrated an increase in IL-5, granulocytemacrophage colony-stimulating factor, and IL-2 in bronchoalveolar lavage fluid in mice exposed to OVA along with sec ondhand smoke. In these mouse models, interferon gamma levels decreased. Because mice exposed to OVA alone did not experience these cytokine changes, secondhand smoke appears able to induce a sensitiza tion phenotype to a usually neutral antigen (Rumold et al. 2001). Although the animal data are stronger than the human epidemiologic data, studies in humans are supportive of an effect of tobacco smoke exposure on allergic phenotypes.

Allergies are caused by multiple interacting factors in people with underlying susceptibility. Secondhand smoke exposure both in utero and after birth may promote the development of an allergic phenotype. Antigens presented during the neonatal period in mice skew the immune development and response along a Th2 pathway (i.e., toward an allergic phenotype) (Forsthuber et al. 1996). Human fetuses, under the influence of the maternal system mediated through the placenta, may develop a Th2 preference as a response to an antigen (Michie 1998). Magnus son (1986) studied newborn children of nonallergic parents and found evidence suggesting that tobacco smoke exposure in utero may promote an aller gic phenotype. A threefold increase in risk for an elevated IgE level was observed in children whose mothers smoked compared with the IgE levels in children born to nonsmoking mothers. Total cord blood IgE concentrations were substantially higher in infants of mothers who smoked (60.8 international units [IU]) compared with infants of nonsmoking mothers (9.8 IU).

Atopy may be characterized by either a positive IgE-mediated skin test or elevated specific IgE serum levels. Atopy represents a risk factor for asthma, and an increase in bronchial responsiveness has been asso ciated with higher serum IgE levels. Human studies provide mixed evidence as to whether secondhand smoke exposures are associated with an increase in IgE-mediated responses (Weiss et al. 1985; Martinez et al. 1988; Ownby and McCullough 1988; Stankus et al. 1988). Weiss and colleagues (1985) demonstrated that maternal smoking was associated with atopy in children aged five through nine years who were eval uated by skin tests to four common allergens. Ron chetti and colleagues (1990) demonstrated an effect of exposure on IgE levels and on eosinophil counts. Eosinophil counts were at least three times higher in boys exposed to secondhand smoke compared with unexposed boys. There was a dose-response relation ship between the number of cigarettes to which each boy had been exposed and the level of eosinophilia (Ronchetti et al. 1990).

Researchers showed decades ago that main stream cigarette smoke causes airway inflammation (Niewoehner et al. 1974) and an increase in airway permeability to small and large molecules in young smokers (Simani et al. 1974; Jones et al. 1980). Given the qualitative similarities between mainstream smoke and secondhand smoke, these effects may be relevant to involuntary smoking (USDHHS 1986).

There are many specific components of second hand smoke that may adversely affect a child's lung. For example, a bacterial endotoxin known as lipopoly saccharide (LPS) can be detected in both mainstream and sidestream tobacco smoke. Studies have detected biologically active LPS in mainstream and sidestream smoke from regular and light experimental refer ence cigarettes used in the studies (mainstream: 120 ± 64 nanograms [ng] per regular cigarette, 45.3 ± 16 ng per light cigarette; sidestream: 18 ± 1.5 ng per regular cigarette, 75 ± 49 ng per light cigarette). The investigators suggested that chronic LPS exposure from cigarette smoke may contribute to the inflamma tory effects of secondhand smoke (Hasday et al. 1999). Other studies show that LPS exposure may alter responses to allergen challenge (Tuli~ et al. 2000).

Researchers need to consider this hypothesized role of endotoxin because of the known pathologic effects of endotoxins on susceptible individuals. As a component of the cell wall of gram-negative bacteria, endotoxins are ubiquitous in the environment and may be found in high concentrations in household dust (Michel et al. 1996) and in ambient air pollution (Bonner et al. 1998). Macrophage activation may result from exposure to low concentrations of an endotoxin, leading to a cascade of inflammatory cytokines (such as IL-1, IL-6, and IL-8) and arachidonic acid metabolites, which are important in the formation of prostaglandin molecules (Bayne et al. 1986; Michie et al. 1988; Ingalls et al. 1999). Studies have documented increased levels of neutrophils in bronchoalveolar lavage fluid after a challenge with dust that contained endotoxins (Hunt et al. 1994). Reversible airflow obstruction has been associated with the inhalation of endotoxins in the air. In a cohort study of infants in Boston, Park and colleagues (2001) used a univariate model and found a significant association of wheeze in the first year of life with elevated dust endotoxin levels (relative risk [RR] = 1.29 [95 percent confidence interval (CI), 1.03–1.62]). In a multivariate model, elevated endo toxin levels in dust were associated with an increased risk for repeated wheeze illness in the first year of life (RR = 1.56 [95 percent CI, 1.03–2.38]) (Park et al. 2001). Exposure to endotoxins from secondhand smoke in utero, during infancy, and in childhood may increase airway inflammation and may interact synergistically with additional secondhand smoke exposures.

Smoking contributes generally to the particulate load in indoor air, and research documents that inhal ing particles in the respirable size range contributes to pulmonary inflammation (National Research Council 2004). One consequence of particle-induced inflamma tion may be an intermediate phenotype with cough and wheeze in early childhood. Investigators used a guinea pig model of secondhand smoke exposure to study sensory nerve pathways for cough and airway narrowing in an effort to explain the development of cough and wheeze symptoms in children of smok ers. When guinea pigs were exposed to sidestream smoke for six hours per day, five days per week, from one through six weeks of age, they demonstrated an increase in excitability of pulmonary C fibers (Mutoh et al. 1999) and rapidly adapting receptors (Bonham et al. 1996), which are believed to be primarily respon sible for eliciting the reflex responses in defending the lungs against inhaled irritants and toxins (Lee and Widdicombe 2001). These studies have led to the con clusion that cough and wheeze may be produced by neural pathway stimulation and irritation.

Summary

Childhood respiratory disease covers a spectrum of diseases and underlying pathogenetic mechanisms that include infection, prenatal alterations in lung structure, inflammation, and allergic responses. There is a potential for secondhand smoke to contribute over the long term to the development of respiratory dis ease through altered organ maturation and immune function. Mechanisms underlying the adverse health effects of secondhand smoke vary across the phases of lung growth and development, extending from the in utero period to the completion of lung growth in late adolescence. The long-term effects of secondhand smoke is a field of ongoing research. These effects may vary among individuals because of individual genetic susceptibilities and gene-environment interactions. The discussions that follow summarize the available observational evidence concerning health effects of secondhand tobacco smoke on children, which are presumed to reflect the mechanisms reviewed above. The discussions also interpret the evidence in the con text of this mechanistic understanding.

METHODS USED TO REVIEW THE EVIDENCE

The search strategies and statistical methods for pooling that were used for this report were identical to those applied to the earlier reviews of this topic car ried out by Strachan and Cook (1997). The authors con ducted an electronic search of the EMBASE Excepta Medica and Medline databases using Medical Subject Headings (MeSH) to select published papers, letters, and review articles relating to secondhand tobacco smoke exposure in children. The EMBASE strategy was based on text word searches of titles, keywords, and related abstracts; non-English language articles were not included. The search was carried out through 2001.

Information relating to the odds ratio (OR) for the outcome of interest among children with and without smokers in the family was extracted from each study. Data regarding children exposed and unexposed to maternal smoking prenatally or post natally were extracted separately. This review also specifically addresses the effects on children of smok ing by other household members (usually the father) when the mother was not a smoker. Not every study provided information on all of these indices. The most common measures were smoking by either parent versus neither parent, and the effects of smoking by the mother versus only by the father or by neither par ent. Few studies distinguished in any detail between prenatal and postnatal maternal smoking, but those that did were included in the discussion. The ORs for the effects of smoking by both parents compared with neither parent were also extracted from cross-sectional surveys of school-age children.

Because most studies have used self-reported parental smoking behaviors as the principal exposure indicator, and because the major sources of exposure in western countries are overwhelmingly maternal fol lowed by paternal smoking (Cook et al. 1994), the terms parental, maternal, and paternal smoking are used throughout this chapter to refer to major sources of secondhand tobacco smoke exposure for children. The OR was chosen as a measure of association because it can be derived from all types of studies—case-control, cross-sectional, and cohort. In general, ORs and their 95 percent CIs were calculated from data in published tabulations using the actual numbers of participants, or numbers estimated from percentages of published column or row totals. This approach allowed for flex ibility in combining categories of household tobacco smoke exposure for comparability across studies.

If the number of participants was not provided, the published OR and its 95 percent CI were used. For some studies, it was necessary to derive an approximate standard error (for the log OR) based on the marginal values of the relevant multiplication table (2×2). In situations where ORs were given separately for different genders, a pooled OR and 95 percent CI were calculated by taking a weighted average (on the log scale) using weights inversely proportional to the variances. The papers that quoted an incidence rate ratio rather than an OR are identified in the summary tabulations.

The literature review also identified information on the extent to which the effects of parental smoking were altered by adjustment for potential confounding variables, and whether there was evidence of an exposure-response relationship with, for example, the amount smoked by either parent. Where the presented data could be standardized for age, gender, or occasionally for another confounder, the Mantel-Haenszel method was used to provide an adjusted value. Because there may be multiple published reports for a single study, only one paper from each study (usually the most recently published) was included in the quantitative meta-analyses. In some studies, however, information from other papers contributed to the assessment of potential confounding or a dose-response relationship.

Updated meta-analyses of the health effects from parental smoking were conducted specifically for this chapter. All pooled estimates were calculated using both fixed and random effects models (Egger et al. 2001). All updated analyses were carried out using Stata. For some outcomes, studies were grouped according to the timing of the secondhand smoke exposure (e.g., maternal smoking during pregnancy, parental smoking from infancy to four years of age, and parental smoking at five or more years of age).

The meta-analysis of the cross-sectional evidence relating parental smoking to spirometric indices in children updates the 1998 meta-analysis (Cook et al. 1998). Both the earlier and the more recent meta analyses used the same effect measure: the average difference in the spirometric index between exposed and unexposed children, expressed as a percentage of the level in the unexposed group. The updated synthesis considered four different spirometric indices: forced vital capacity (FVC), forced expiratory volume in one second (FEV1), mid-expiratory flow rate (MEFR), and flow rates at end expiration. Pooled estimates of the percentage differences were calculated using both fixed and random effects models (Egger et al. 2001).

To determine whether the exposure classification influenced the relationship between parental smoking and lung function, studies were pooled within the following exposure groups: both parents did versus did not smoke, mother did versus did not smoke, either parent versus neither parent smoked, the highest versus the lowest cotinine category, and high levels of household secondhand smoke versus none. To test for effects on the relationship between parental smoking and lung function from adjustment for variables other than age, gender, and body size, studies were pooled separately depending on adjustment for other variables. Lastly, this meta-analysis also assessed whether adjusting for socioeconomic measures, such as parental education and social class, affected the pooled results.

LOWER RESPIRATORY ILLNESSES IN INFANCY AND EARLY CHILDHOOD

This section summarizes the evidence relating specifically to acute LRIs in the first two or three years of life and updates the previous review by Strachan and Cook (1997). Separate discussions review studies of asthma incidence, prognosis, and severity as well as studies (mostly cross-sectional) of school-age children.

In developed countries, the specific microbial etiology and determinants of some common lower respiratory tract illnesses in infancy remain a subject of uncertainty and research (Silverman 1993; Wilson 1994; Monto 2002; Klig and Chen 2003). Although many LRIs result from viral infections, there is an indication of a prenatally determined susceptibility related to lung function abnormalities that is already detectable at birth (Dezateux and Stocks 1997). As reviewed in the introduction to this chapter, lasting effects of in utero exposure to tobacco smoke from maternal smoking may increase airway resistance and the likelihood of a more severe LRI with infection.

This review covers the full spectrum of LRIs, include ing categories considered to reflect infection and the category of wheeze, which may be a consequence of infection but may also indicate an asthma phenotype.

There is also an emerging consensus that there are several phenotypes of childhood wheeze, each with a different pattern of incidence, prognosis, and risk factors (Wilson 1994; Christie and Helms 1995).

However, there is much less certainty about how these different "asthma phenotypes" should be character ized for either research or clinical purposes.

Findings from the Tucson (Arizona) birth cohort study suggest physiologic and immunologic differences between the phenotypic syndromes of early childhood wheeze, the onset of asthma symptoms later in childhood, and persistent disease (Martinez et al. 1995; Stein et al. 1997). These findings have yet to be replicated in a comprehensive way in other large population samples, and few large cohort studies are in progress that pro vide the needed longitudinal data. The classification of phenotype in the epidemiologic studies is relevant to secondhand smoke if the association of secondhand smoke with risk varies across the phenotypes.

Evidence Synthesis

The finding of an association between parental smoking and LRI is consistent across diverse study populations and study designs, methods of case ascer tainment, and diagnostic groupings. The association cannot be attributed to confounding or publication bias. Only two studies found an inverse association. One small study that reported an inverse association for maternal smoking had wide confidence limits and a positive association with cotinine levels in meconium (Nuesslein et al. 1999). A study from Brazil found an inverse association with pneumonia (Victora et al. 1994). Studies in developing countries generally have tended not to find an increased risk associated with exposure of infants and children to parental smoking. This pattern may reflect the different nature of LRIs in developing countries where bacteria are key patho gens and there is a powerful effect from biomass fuel combustion (Smith et al. 2000; Black and Michaelsen 2002), and where levels of secondhand smoke expo sure are possibly lower because of housing character istics and smoking patterns.

Some variation among studies in the magnitude of OR estimates would be anticipated as patterns of smoking differed among countries and over time, and the methods of the studies were not consistent in all respects. This variation is reflected in statistically sig nificant heterogeneity in some of the pooled analyses.

For this reason, the summary ORs derived under the fixed effects assumption should be interpreted with caution. The random effects method may be more appropriate in these circumstances because its wider confidence limits reflect the heterogeneity between studies. This method is, however, more susceptible to the effects of any publication bias because the ran dom effects method gives greater weight to smaller studies. Thus, considering the largest studies only, the fixed effects estimate for maternal smoking was 1.56 and the random effects estimate was 1.72.

Regardless, the pooled estimates were statistically significant and it is highly unlikely that the association emerged by chance.

The papers that have been cited were selected using keywords relevant to passive/involuntary smoking and children in the title or abstract. When cross-checked against previous reviews of involuntary smoking in children, major omissions were not identified (USDHHS 1986; USEPA 1992; DiFranza and Lew 1996; Li et al. 1999), whereas the systematic search identified relevant references not cited elsewhere. There is a possibility that the selection was biased toward studies reporting a positive association; it is more likely that statistically significant findings would be mentioned in the abstract in comparison with nonsignificant or null findings. Three of the higher ORs were derived from small case-control studies in which involuntary smoking was not the focus of the original research (Hall et al. 1984; McConnochie and Roghmann 1986; Hayes et al. 1989), and for these three studies publication bias may have been operative. The slightly higher pooled ORs obtained by the random effects compared with the fixed effects method reflect the greater weight assigned by the random effects approach to these small studies with a relatively large OR. However, inclusion of the large Chinese studies (Chen et al. 1988a; Jin and Rossignol 1993; Chen 1994) in the meta-analysis of the effects of smoking by either parent would have had a conservative effect (i.e., a smaller pooled estimate), because few mothers smoked in these communities.

The biologic basis for the association of paternal smoking with LRI is possibly complex, and may reflect mechanisms of injury that are in play before and after birth. These mechanisms operate to make respiratory infections more severe or to possibly increase the likelihood of infection. Although viral infection is a well-characterized etiologic factor (Graham 1990), there is evidence that the severity of the illness may be determined in part by lung function abnormalities detectable from birth that result from maternal smoking during pregnancy (Dezateux and Stocks 1997). Many early childhood episodes of wheeze, including bronchiolitis, probably form part of this spectrum of viral illnesses, although other episodes may be the first evidence of more persistent childhood asthma with associated atopic manifestations (Silverman 1993; Martinez et al. 1995). The evidence does not indicate that parental smoking increases the rate of infection with respiratory pathogens. Respiratory viruses are isolated with equal frequency among infants in smoking and nonsmoking households (Gardner et al. 1984).

The effect of parental smoking on the incidence of wheeze and nonwheeze illnesses appears similar, suggesting a general increase in susceptibility to clinical illness upon exposure to respiratory infections rather than to influences on mechanisms more specifically related to asthma.

The pooled results from families with nonsmoking mothers suggest that the effects of parental smoking are at least partly attributable to postnatal (i.e., environmental) exposure to tobacco smoke in the home. The somewhat stronger effects of smoking by the mother compared with other household members may be related to the role of the mother as the principal caregiver, which would explain a higher degree of postnatal exposure of the child from the mother's smoking. However, there is also evidence pointing to altered intrauterine lung development as a specific adverse effect of maternal smoking during pregnancy (Tager et al. 1993).

The effect of parental smoking is largely independent of potential confounding variables in studies that have measured and incorporated such variables into the analyses, suggesting that residual confounding by other factors is unlikely. It thus appears that smoking by the parents, rather than characteristics of the family related to smoking, adversely affect children and cause LRIs. The evidence supports the conclusion found in other recent reviews that there is a causal relationship between parental smoking and acute LRIs (USDHHS 1986; USEPA 1992; DiFranza and Lew 1996; WHO 1997; Li et al. 1999; California EPA 2005). The findings are consistent, properly temporal in the exposure-outcome relationship, and biologically plausible. The evidence is strongest for the first two years of life. The studies that were reviewed also suggest a clear reduction in the estimated effect after two to three years of age, particularly for pneumonia and bronchitis. The failure to find statistically significant associations in some studies of older children should not be interpreted, however, as indicative of no effect of secondhand smoke exposure at older ages.

Conclusions

1. The evidence is sufficient to infer a causal relationship between secondhand smoke exposure from parental smoking and lower respiratory illnesses in infants and children.
2. The increased risk for lower respiratory illnesses is greatest from smoking by the mother.

Implications

Respiratory infections remain a leading cause of childhood morbidity in the United States and other developed countries and are a leading cause of childhood deaths worldwide. The effect of parental smoking, particularly maternal smoking, is of a substantial magnitude. Reducing smoking by parents, beginning with maternal smoking during pregnancy, should reduce the occurrence of LRI. Health care practitioners providing care for pregnant women, infants, and children should urge smoking cessation; parents who are unable to quit should be encouraged not to smoke in the home.

MIDDLE EAR DISEASE AND ADENOTONSILLECTOMY

A possible link between parental smoking and the risk of otitis media (OM) with effusion (OME) in children was first suggested in 1983 (Kraemer et al. 1983). A number of subsequent epidemiologic studies have investigated the association of secondhand tobacco smoke exposure with diseases of the ear, nose, and throat (ENT), and the evidence has been summarized in narrative reviews (USEPA 1992; Gulya 1994; Blakley and Blakley 1995; NCI 1999) and quantitative meta-analyses (DiFranza and Lew 1996; Uhari et al. 1996). Strachan and Cook (1998a) systematically reviewed the evidence relating parental smoking to acute otitis media (AOM), recurrent otitis media (ROM), OME (glue ear), and ENT surgery in children. This section updates that 1998 review following the methods described earlier. Full journal publications cited in an overview by Thornton and Lee (1999) were also considered, but abstracts and conference proceedings were not included.

Evidence Synthesis

Evidence from different study designs and for different chronic or recurrent disease outcomes related to the middle ear in young children is remarkably consistent in showing a modest elevation in risk associated with parental smoking. Although the outcome measures used are subject to misclassification, the evidence is nonetheless consistent in spite of this heterogeneity.

Subsequent publications over the last four years have not substantially affected the findings of the 1997 meta-analysis (Strachan and Cook 1998a), although quantitative summarization can now be extended to AOM. No single study addresses all of the potential methodologic concerns about selection (referral) bias, information (reporting) bias, or confounding. However, multiple studies that have considered these potential methodologic problems using objective measurements, matched designs, or multivariate analyses have found that the association of secondhand smoke exposure with middle ear disease persists with little alteration in the magnitude of the effect across stud ies, or within studies that controlled for potential con founding. There are multiple potential pathogenetic mechanisms related to the effects of tobacco smoke components on the upper airway (Samet 2004) (see also Chapter 2, Toxicology of Secondhand Smoke in the full report). A causal association between acute and chronic middle ear disease and secondhand smoke exposure is thus biologically plausible.

Conclusions

1. The evidence is sufficient to infer a causal relationship between parental smoking and middle ear disease in children, including acute and recurrent otitis media and chronic middle ear effusion.
2. The evidence is suggestive but not sufficient to infer a causal relationship between parental smoking and the natural history of middle ear effusion.
3. The evidence is inadequate to infer the presence or absence of a causal relationship between parental smoking and an increase in the risk of adenoidectomy or tonsillectomy among children.

Implications

The etiology of acute and chronic middle ear disease is still a focus of investigation. Nonetheless, the finding that parental smoking causes middle ear disease offers an opportunity for the prevention of this common problem. Health care providers making diagnoses of acute and chronic middle ear disease need to communicate with parents who smoke con cerning the consequences for their children.

RESPIRATORY SYMPTOMS AND PREVALENT ASTHMA IN SCHOOL-AGE CHILDREN

The first reports (based on telephone surveys) documenting an adverse effect of parental smoking on the health of children were published in the late 1960s (Cameron 1967; Cameron et al. 1969). By the early 1970s, studies with more formal designs addressed respiratory symptoms (Norman-Taylor and Dickin son

1972; Colley 1974; Colley et al. 1974). Since then, many epidemiologic studies have found an association between parental smoking and respiratory symptoms and diseases throughout childhood. These outcomes were considered in the 1984 and 1986 reports of the Surgeon General (USDHHS 1984, 1986). The narrative review of the 1992 EPA risk assessment (USEPA 1992) concluded that the evidence causally relating secondhand smoke exposure at home to respiratory symptoms was very strong among preschool-age children, but less compelling in school-age children. A subsequent quantitative review did not distinguish between different types of secondhand smoke exposure and their effects at different ages (DiFranza and Lew 1996).

This section summarizes the evidence on the prevalence of respiratory symptoms and asthma in children aged 5 through 16 years, assessed from surveys carried out in schools or populations. This review includes primarily cross-sectional studies and cohorts studied at a single point in time, and updates an earlier 1997 review by Cook and Strachan (1997). A subsequent section of this chapter addresses studies on the onset of asthma and exposure to secondhand smoke. These two sets of outcome measures for asthma—prevalent and incident disease—were separated because disease prevalence reflects not only factors determining incidence, but factors affecting persistence. The studies of asthma prevalence, however, receive further consideration when assessing the evidence related to asthma onset. There are additional complexities in comparisons across studies of varied designs that arise from the different approaches used to ascertain the presence of asthma, and from the heterogeneity of the asthma phenotype by age. Additionally, wheeze, cough, phlegm, and breathlessness are common symptoms for children with asthma.

Evidence Synthesis

This report has described multiple mechanisms by which secondhand smoke exposure could increase the prevalence of respiratory symptoms and asthma in childhood. Secondhand smoke exposure might increase the prevalence of respiratory symptoms and asthma through in utero effects or through inflammation and an altered lung immunophenotype from postnatal exposure. Multiple studies from diverse countries consistently show that parental smoking is positively associated with the prevalence of asthma and respiratory symptoms (including wheeze) in schoolchildren; the findings of individual studies as well as the pooled analyses show that these associations are unlikely to be attributable to chance alone. The magnitude of the effects is similar for the different outcome measures. The estimated effects, particularly for wheeze, were robust to adjustments for a wide range of potentially confounding environmental and other factors. This robustness supports the conclusion that residual confounding is unlikely to be an issue and that the associations between parental smoking and the prevalence of asthma and respiratory symptoms in schoolchildren are causal.

The case for a causal interpretation is further strengthened by the trend for the OR to increase with the number of parents who smoke (i.e., none, one, or both). In the meta-analysis, the trends with the number of smoking parents were statistically significant for asthma, wheeze, and cough, and trends were evident in most of the individual studies as well. The effect of maternal smoking is greater than that of paternal smoking, but there is nevertheless evidence for a small effect of paternal smoking. Maternal smoking is associated with higher cotinine levels in school-age children, implying that maternal smoking probably has a greater impact on the exposure of children to secondhand smoke (Cook et al. 1994). These results also imply that the increased risk for asthma and other symptoms reflects postnatal exposure, although prenatal exposure may also be a contributing factor. First, there is an effect of paternal smoking; second, risk tends to rise with the number of household smokers; third, many women who do not smoke while pregnant smoke after the birth of their children; and fourth, limited evidence shows no increase in symptoms in children of former smokers. Few studies have examined dose-response trends with the number of cigarettes smoked in the household per day or dose-response trends among exposed children alone.

The prevalence of symptoms ascertained by cross-sectional surveys is determined by both disease incidence and prognosis, and the pattern of morbidity tends to be dominated by a large number of children with mild symptoms. There are indications that secondhand smoke exposure is associated with more severe wheeze, both in studies where ORs were reported for different severity measures and in studies where ORs were highest when the prevalence of wheeze was low.

Conclusions

1. The evidence is sufficient to infer a causal relationship between parental smoking and cough, phlegm, wheeze, and breathlessness among children of school age.
2. The evidence is sufficient to infer a causal relationship between parental smoking and ever having asthma among children of school age.

Implications

Respiratory symptoms are common among children, even among those without asthma. Second hand smoke exposure increases the risk for the major symptoms; these symptoms should not be dismissed as minor because they may impact the activities of the affected children. Secondhand smoke exposure is causally associated with asthma prevalence, perhaps reflecting a greater clinical severity associated with exposure. Secondhand smoke exposure, particularly at home, should be addressed by clinicians caring for any child with a respiratory complaint and particu larly children with asthma.

CHILDHOOD ASTHMA ONSET

As discussed earlier in this chapter (see "Lower Respiratory Illnesses in Infancy and Early Child hood"), parental smoking is causally associated with an increased incidence of acute LRIs, including ill nesses with wheeze, in the first one or two years of a child's life. Prevalence surveys of schoolchildren show that wheeze and diagnosed asthma are more common among children of smoking parents, with a greater elevation in risk for outcomes based on definitions of wheeze that reflect a greater severity. Evidence pre sented in the prior section supported conclusions that parental smoking was causally associated with respi ratory symptoms and prevalent asthma; the cross- sectional evidence did not address asthma onset. This section reviews cohort and case-control studies of wheeze illnesses that provide evidence concerning the effects of parental smoking on the incidence, prog nosis, and severity of childhood asthma. The design of these studies addresses the temporal relationship between exposure and disease onset. This discussion also considers case-control studies of prevalent asthma that provide findings complementary to the surveys of schoolchildren. This section represents an update of the 1998 review by Strachan and Cook (1998c).

Evidence Synthesis

The results summarized in this discussion and in previous sections present a complex picture of the associations of parental smoking with asthma inci dence, prognosis, prevalence, and severity. The rates of incidence and recurrence of wheeze illnesses in early life are greater if there is smoking in the home, particularly by the mother, whereas the incidence of asthma during the school-age years is less strongly affected by parental smoking. A similar age-related decline in the strength of the effect of secondhand smoke exposure is evident in cross-sectional studies. These findings may simply reflect the diminishing level of secondhand tobacco smoke exposure from household sources as children age (Irvine et al. 1997; Chang et al. 2000). Alternatively or additionally, parental smoking may have differential effects on the incidence of various forms of wheeze illnesses; there may be a stronger effect on the viral infection associated with wheeze that is common in early childhood, and a weaker effect on the atopic wheeze that occurs often as a later onset component of asthma (Wilson 1989). Five studies comparing the effect of smoking on wheeze in atopic and nonatopic children lend support to the latter hypothesis (Kershaw 1987; Palmieri et al. 1990; Chen et al. 1996; Strachan et al. 1996; Rönmark et al. 1999), but a sixth does not (Murray and Morrison 1990).

The earlier section on LRIs in infancy presented evidence of an increased risk from postnatal exposure to smoking by the father in households where the mother did not smoke, but there was insufficient evidence to distinguish the separate effects of prenatal and postnatal smoking by the mother. Several of the cohort studies reviewed here have reported findings in relation to maternal smoking during pregnancy. These data are limited, and the potential role of prenatal exposure as an independent cause of asthma is still unclear. The published data are insufficient to assess the independent effect of nonmaternal smoking on the incidence or natural history of childhood asthma after the first few years of life. Most cohort studies show a weak association of asthma incidence with paternal smoking. In case-control studies, maternal smoking has the dominant effect, with little effect from smoking by the father.

Although wheeze in infancy is more likely to recur if both parents smoke, at least maternal smoking alone is associated with seemingly little long-term risk. This indication could also reflect a stronger association of parental smoking with nonatopic wheeze ("wheezy bronchitis" than with "allergic asthma"), which is associated with a better prognosis. On the other hand, atopic children tend to have more severe and more frequent or persistent wheeze, and case-control studies of ("clinic") children with more severe asthma show a positive association with maternal smoking that again appears to be of greater importance. Indeed, the pooled OR for smoking by either parent from these case-control studies (1.39) is somewhat greater than the corresponding pooled ORs from cross-sectional surveys of wheeze (1.27) and asthma (1.22) among schoolchildren. Furthermore, most studies have found a greater severity of disease among children with asthma if the parents smoke, and prevalence surveys among schoolchildren suggest a stronger association with more restrictive (presumably more severe) definitions of wheeze than with any recent wheeze.

These findings by age and phenotype are complex to interpret: studies of incidence and prognosis suggest an association of parental smoking primarily with early, nonatopic wheeze that tends to run a mild and transient course, whereas studies of prevalence and severity suggest that secondhand tobacco smoke exposure increases the risk of more severe symptoms and more outpatient clinic visits or emergency hospital admissions. One explanation for this pattern would be to consider secondhand tobacco smoke as a cofactor operating with intercurrent infections as a trigger of wheeze attacks, rather than as a factor initiating or inducing persistent asthma. This distinction between induction (initiation) and exacerbation (provocation) also emerges when considering the role of outdoor air pollution as a cause of asthma (Department of Health Committee on the Medical Effects of Air Pollutants 1995). There is also strong familial aggregation for childhood asthma that certainly has genetic determinants, although research on the genetics of asthma is still inconclusive.

The incidence of both wheeze and nonwheeze LRIs in infancy increases to a similar extent if both parents smoke, and the increase reflects, at least in part, postnatal secondhand (environmental) tobacco smoke exposure. It is likely that the clinical severity of viral respiratory infections in older children is also exacerbated by secondhand smoke exposure, which leads to an increased risk of respiratory symptoms in general, including wheeze. Among children at low risk for wheeze, secondhand smoke exposure at the time of an intercurrent infection may be sufficient to cause occasional episodes of asthmatic symptoms and thus increase the risk of a mild, often transient wheeze tendency that the child outgrows as the airways become larger or less reactive with increasing age. In a previous section of this chapter, the conclusion was reached that secondhand smoke exposure from parental smoking causes LRIs in infants and children. The wheezing that accompanies many of these LRIs may be clinically classified as asthma, although the cohort study findings suggest that this phenotype is not generally persistent as the child ages.

Some previous reviews have concluded that exposure to secondhand smoke is causally associated with an increase in the incidence of childhood asthma (USEPA 1992; Halken et al. 1995). This association has been attributed to chronic (but possibly reversible) effects of parental smoking on bronchial hyperreactivity rather than to the acute effects of cigarette smoke on airway caliber (USEPA 1992). The most relevant evidence for secondhand smoke exposure and onset of asthma comes from studies of older children at an age when there is reasonable diagnostic certainty. This evidence comes from only a small number of studies and their statistical power is limited, particularly within specific age strata. In addition, all studies are inherently limited by the difficulty of classifying the outcome, and there may be variations in the phenotypes that were considered across the studies. Within these constraints, the evidence indicating an association of secondhand smoke exposure from parental smoking with asthma incidence is inconsistent. The evidence for asthma prevalence, by contrast, was sufficient to support an inference of causality.

Conclusions

1. The evidence is sufficient to infer a causal relationship between secondhand smoke exposure from parental smoking and the onset of wheeze illnesses in early childhood.
2. The evidence is suggestive but not sufficient to infer a causal relationship between secondhand smoke exposure from parental smoking and the onset of childhood asthma.

Implications

The etiology of childhood asthma includes the interplay of genetic and environmental factors. The asthma phenotype likely comprises several distinct entities. The evidence is clear in showing that secondhand smoke exposure causes wheeze illnesses in early life and makes asthma more severe clinically. This evidence provides a strong basis for limiting exposure of infants and children to secondhand smoke, even though a causal link with asthma onset is not yet established for asthma incidence.

ATOPY

The hypothesis that secondhand tobacco smoke exposure might increase allergic sensitization was first proposed more than 20 years ago (Kjellman 1981). However, the role of secondhand smoke exposure (specifically from maternal smoking) in allergic sensitization remains uncertain despite many investigations since that time. Some studies have documented an association between maternal smoking during pregnancy and elevated cord blood total IgE, as well as an elevated risk for the development of allergic disease (Magnusson 1986; Bergmann et al. 1995). Other studies, however, have not replicated these findings (Halonen et al. 1991; Oryszczyn et al. 1991; Ownby et al. 1991). Many studies have investigated the relationships of secondhand smoke exposure from parental smoking with cord blood IgE concentrations, IgE levels later in childhood, skin-test reactivity, and allergic manifestations such as rhinitis (Strachan and Cook 1998c). The comprehensive, systematic review reported by Strachan and Cook (1998c) of the effects of secondhand smoke exposure from parental smoking covered IgE levels, skin-prick test reactivity, and allergic rhinitis and eczema. The review included 9 studies of IgE levels in neonates, 8 studies of IgE levels in older children, 12 studies of skin-prick tests, and 10 studies of allergic symptoms (Strachan and Cook 1998c). The quantitative summary did not show a significant association of maternal smoking with total serum IgE, allergic rhinitis, or eczema. The meta-analysis for skin-prick test positivity and smoking during infancy and pregnancy yielded a pooled OR estimate of 0.87 (95 percent CI, 0.62–1.24), suggesting no effect of secondhand smoke on skin-prick positivity during these stages of development. The summary estimate supported a conclusion that maternal smoking before birth or parental smoking during infancy is unlikely to increase the risk of allergic sensitization.

This conclusion remains consistent with results from studies conducted since this systematic review, which also found no increase in risk for allergic sensitization from secondhand smoke exposure. The discussion that follows reviews some of the key studies published since 1997.

Evidence Synthesis

There are multiple mechanisms by which secondhand smoke exposure might alter the risk for allergic diseases in infants and children. Exposure to tobacco smoke components from maternal smoking during pregnancy might have lasting effects on lung and systemic immunophenotypes. Exposures after birth might also affect immunophenotype or increase susceptibility to sensitization by common allergens.

The observational evidence across a range of outcome measures is inconsistent, however. The inconsistency may partially reflect the limited number of studies for any particular outcome and the methodologic complexities of studies on atopic disorders.

Conclusion

1. The evidence is inadequate to infer the presence or absence of a causal relationship between parental smoking and the risk of immunoglobulin E-mediated allergy in their children.

Implications

Studies on secondhand smoke exposure and atopy need to be prospective in design and should track exposures back to the pregnancy. Further stud ies on secondhand smoke and atopy in childhood are needed, but the studies need to be large enough and need to have sufficient and valid measurements of allergic phenotype. Future studies also need to address potential genetic determinants of susceptibil ity, particularly as they modify the effect of second hand smoke.

LUNG GROWTH AND PULMONARY FUNCTION

Beginning with the 1984 report (USDHHS 1984), the U.S. Surgeon General's reports in this series have covered the adverse effects of exposure to second hand smoke, including effects from maternal smoking during pregnancy and effects on lung growth from exposure during infancy and childhood. Both cross- sectional and cohort studies on this topic have used lung function level as the primary indicator. The level of lung function achieved at any particular age and measured cross-sectionally is an indicator of the rate of growth of function up to that age; cohort studies with repeated measurements of lung function directly esti mate the rate of growth. The 1986 Surgeon General's report, *The Health Consequences of Involuntary Smoking,* reviewed 18 cross-sectional and cohort studies and concluded that "available data demonstrate that maternal smoking reduced lung function in young children" (USDHHS 1986, p. 54). The report further suggests that although this reduction is small, with an average of 1 to 5 percent, "some children might be affected to a greater extent, and even small differ ences might be important for children who become active cigarette smokers as adults" (USDHHS 1986, p. 54). The EPA issued its risk assessment in 1992 and concluded that the decline in lung function associated with exposure to secondhand smoke represented a causal effect (USEPA 1992). Similar conclusions were reached by the California Environmental Protection Agency (NCI 1999) and WHO (1999). Thus, for nearly two decades the weight of evidence has been sufficient to conclude that prenatal and postnatal tobacco smoke exposure is associated with a decrease in lung func tion in childhood. As discussed earlier in this chapter (see "Mechanisms of Health Effects from Secondhand Tobacco Smoke"), lung maturation and growth decre ments secondary to exposure are reflected in changes in measured pulmonary function.

A 1998 meta-analysis by Cook and colleagues (1998) concluded that maternal smoking was associ ated with reduced ventilatory function assessed by spirometry. In a quantitative synthesis of 21 cross- sectional studies, the effects of parental smoking on lung function were reductions of the FVC by 0.2 per cent (95 percent CI, -0.4–0.1), the FEV1 by 0.9 percent (95 percent CI, -1.2 to -0.7), the MEFR by 4.8 percent (95 percent CI, -5.4 to -4.3), and the end-expiratory flow rate (EEFR) by 4.3 percent (95 percent CI, -5.3 to -3.3). The meta-analysis also considered six prospec tive cohort studies and found only a small effect of current exposure on decreased growth in lung func tion. The researchers attributed most of the decreased growth to a lasting consequence of in utero exposure from maternal smoking (Cook et al. 1998).

This discussion considers some of the studies included in this 1998 meta-analysis in addition to studies published subsequently. The studies are both cross-sectional and cohort in design, include data on maternal smoking during pregnancy and after birth, and indicate that maternal smoking during pregnancy has a substantially greater adverse effect. As discussed above, maternal smoking affects lung development in utero perhaps by a direct toxic effect, by gene regu lation, or by leading to developmental abnormalities. The number of airways in the lung is considered fixed by the time a child is born, but the number of alveoli in the lung increases until four years of age (Dezateux and Stocks 1997). The period from gestation to four years of age thus represents a vulnerable time for lung growth and development, and exposures during this time are potentially the most critical for structural and functional lung development and performance. This section reviews the evidence that associates different phases of lung growth and development with corre sponding ages.

Evidence Synthesis

Smoking during pregnancy exposes the develop ing lung to a variety of toxins and reduces the delivery of oxygen to the fetus (USDHHS 2001). Animal mod els indicate structural consequences that may under lie the physiologic effects that are well documented shortly after birth. Secondhand smoke exposure from parents who smoke would be expected to lead to pulmonary inflammation that would be sustained across childhood.

Thus, there is substantial biologic plausibility for causation of reduced lung growth by secondhand smoke exposure. Multiple studies have measured lung function shortly after birth and document the adverse effects on lung function from maternal smoking during pregnancy. The pattern of abnormalities is suggestive of a persistent adverse effect on the airways of the fetus from maternal smoking during pregnancy.

There is also substantial evidence from both cross-sectional and cohort studies of a sustained effect from in utero exposure, as well as an additional adverse effect from postnatal exposure. Multiple studies have shown cumulative consequences of both prenatal and postnatal exposures. Across the set of studies, potentially important confounding factors have been given consideration and the adverse effects of secondhand smoke exposure on lung function cannot be attributed to other factors.

In the context of this body of evidence against causal criteria, the effects of prenatal and postnatal exposures merit separate consideration because they correspond to substantially different phases of development and potential susceptibility. For both exposures, the evidence is substantial and consistent. There are multiple bases for biologic plausibility, and the temporal relationships of exposures with the outcome measures are appropriate.

Conclusions

1. The evidence is sufficient to infer a causal relationship between maternal smoking during pregnancy and persistent adverse effects on lung function across childhood.

2. The evidence is sufficient to infer a causal relationship between exposure to secondhand smoke after birth and a lower level of lung function during childhood.

Implications

Lung growth continues throughout childhood and adolescence and is completed by young adulthood, when lung growth peaks and then begins to decline as a result of aging, smoking, and other environmental factors. The evidence shows that parental smoking reduces the maximum achieved level, although not to a degree (on average) that would impair individuals. Nonetheless, a reduced peak level increases the risk for future chronic lung disease, and there is heterogeneity of the effect so that some exposed children may have a much greater reduction than the mean. In addition, children of smokers are more likely to become smokers and thus face a future risk for impairment from active smoking.

CONCLUSIONS

The following conclusions are supported by text in the full report that may not be included in this excerpt. The full report can be accessed at http://www.surgeongeneral.gov/library/second handsmoke/report/.

Lower Respiratory Illnesses in Infancy and Early Childhood

1. The evidence is sufficient to infer a causal relationship between secondhand smoke exposure from parental smoking and lower respiratory illnesses in infants and children.

2 The increased risk for lower respiratory illnesses is greatest from smoking by the mother.

Middle Ear Disease and Adenotonsillectomy

3. The evidence is sufficient to infer a causal relationship between parental smoking and middle ear disease in children, including acute and recurrent otitis media and chronic middle ear effusion.

4. The evidence is suggestive but not sufficient to infer a causal relationship between parental smoking and the natural history of middle ear effusion.

5. The evidence is inadequate to infer the presence or absence of a causal relationship between parental smoking and an increase in the risk of adenoidectomy or tonsillectomy among children.

Respiratory Symptoms and Prevalent Asthma in School-Age Children

6. The evidence is sufficient to infer a causal relationship between parental smoking and cough, phlegm, wheeze, and breathlessness among children of school age.

7. The evidence is sufficient to infer a causal relationship between parental smoking and ever having asthma among children of school age.

Childhood Asthma Onset

8. The evidence is sufficient to infer a causal relationship between secondhand smoke exposure from parental smoking and the onset of wheeze illnesses in early childhood.
9. The evidence is suggestive but not sufficient to infer a causal relationship between secondhand smoke exposure from parental smoking and the onset of childhood asthma.

Lung Growth and Pulmonary Function

10. The evidence is sufficient to infer a causal relationship between maternal smoking during pregnancy and persistent adverse effects on lung function across childhood.
11. The evidence is sufficient to infer a causal relationship between exposure to secondhand smoke after birth and a lower level of lung function during childhood.

Atopy

12. The evidence is inadequate to infer the presence or absence of a causal relationship between parental smoking and the risk of immunoglobulin E-mediated allergy in their children.

OVERALL IMPLICATIONS

The extensive evidence considered in this chapter causally links parental smoking to adverse health effects in children. The association between parental smoking and childhood respiratory disease is stronger at younger ages, a pattern plausibly explained by a higher level of exposure to secondhand smoke among infants and preschool-age children for any given level of parental smoking. In general, associations with maternal smoking are stronger than with paternal smoking, but for several outcomes, associations were found for smoking by the father in homes where the mother does not smoke. This finding argues strongly for an independent adverse effect of a post natal involuntary (environmental) exposure to second hand smoke in the home. There may be an additional hazard related to prenatal exposure of the fetus to maternal smoking during pregnancy (USDHHS 2001, 2004). The published evidence does not adequately separate the independent effects on childhood respi ratory health of prenatal versus postnatal exposure to maternal smoking. This unresolved research issue should not detract from the public health message that smoking by either parent is potentially damaging to the health of children.

Interpretation of the evidence is perhaps most complex in relation to childhood asthma, which is a term generally applied to a mixed group of clinical phenotypes. Recurrent wheeze illnesses are common among young children, and there is controversy about whether these illnesses should all be classified as "asthma." Cohort studies show that symptoms do not persist for many children beyond the first few years of life. The balance of evidence strongly sup ports a causal relationship between parental smoking and the incidence of wheeze illnesses in infancy, the prevalence of wheeze and related symptoms among schoolchildren, and the relative severity of disease among children with physician-diagnosed asthma. These are all important indicators of a substantial and potentially preventable public health burden.

The evidence related to the wheeze illnesses can be separated to an extent from that related to a clearer clinical phenotype of asthma, a chronic condi tion of variable airflow obstruction with a heightened susceptibility to environmental triggers of broncho spasm. The evidence is less clear as to whether paren tal smoking initiates the disease among previously healthy children. Because the clinical diagnosis of asthma relies to a large extent upon a history of recur rent wheeze attacks or other chest illnesses, any expo sure (including parental smoking) that increases the incidence of such episodes will tend to be associated with an apparent increase in the incidence of diag nosed "asthma," even if secondhand smoke exposure does not contribute to the incidence directly. Studies of nonspecific bronchial responsiveness, a surrogate for the asthma phenotype, offer some insights into the long-term susceptibility that underlies chronic asthma. Secondhand smoke exposure is linked to an increase in responsiveness, beginning with in utero exposure. However, bronchial responsiveness is also nonspecifi cally and transiently increased following respiratory tract infections. For this reason, the conclusion regard ing parental smoking as a cause of childhood asthma has been phrased in less definite terms than the con clusions relating to asthma prevalence and severity.

REFERENCES

Barker K, Mussin E, Taylor DK. Fetal exposure to involuntary maternal smoking and childhood respiratory disease. *Annals of Allergy, Asthma, and Immunology.* 1996;76(5):427–30.

Bayne EK, Rupp EA, Limjuco G, Chin J, Schmidt JA. Immunocytochemical detection of interleukin 1 within stimulated human monocytes. *Journal of Experimental Medicine.* 1986;163(5):1267–80.

Bergmann RL, Schulz J, Gunther S, Dudenhausen JW, Bergmann KE, Bauer CP, Dorsch W, Schmidt E, Luck W, Lau S. Determinants of cord-blood IgE concentrations in 6401 German neonates. *Allergy.* 1995;50(1):65–71.

Black RE, Michaelsen KF. *Public Health Issues in Infant and Child Nutrition.* Philadelphia: Lippincott Wil liams and Wilkins, 2002.

Blakley BW, Blakley JE. Smoking and middle ear disease: are they related? A review arti cle. *Otolaryngology—Head and Neck Surgery.* 1995;112(3):441–6.

Bonham AC, Kott KS, Joad JP. Sidestream smoke expo sure enhances rapidly adapting receptor responses to substance P in young guinea pigs. *Journal of Applied Physiology.* 1996;81(4):1715–22.

Bonner JC, Rice AB, Lindroos PM, O'Brien PO, Dreher KL, Rosas I, Alfaro-Moreno E, Osornio-Vargas AR. Induction of the lung myofibroblast PDGF receptor system by urban ambient particles from Mexico City. *American Journal of Respiratory Cell and Molecular Biology.* 1998;19(4):672–80.

Braun KM, Cornish T, Valm A, Cundiff J, Pauly JL, Fan S. Immunotoxicology of cigarette smoke condensates: suppression of macrophage respon siveness to interferon -γ. *Toxicology and Applied Pharmacology.* 1998;149(2):136–43.

Brown RW, Hanrahan JP, Castile RG, Tager IB. Effect of maternal smoking during pregnancy on passive respiratory mechanics in early infancy. *Pediatric Pulmonology.* 1995;19(1):23–8.

California Environmental Protection Agency. *Proposed Identification of Environmental Tobacco Smoke as a Toxic Air Contaminant. Part B: Health Effects.* Sacramento (CA): California Environmental Pro tection Agency, Office of Environmental Health Hazard Assessment, 2005.

Cameron P. The presence of pets and smoking as correlates of perceived disease. *Journal of Allergy* 1967;40(1):12–5.

Cameron P, Kostin JS, Zaks JM, Wolfe JH, Tighe G, Oselett B, Stocker R, Winton J. The health of smokers' and non-smokers' children. *Journal of Allergy.* 1969;43(6):336–41.

Catlin EA, Powell SM, Manganaro TF, Hudson PL, Ragin RC, Epstein J, Donahoe PK. Sex-specific fetal lung development and Müllerian inhibiting substance. *American Review of Respiratory Diseases.* 1990;141(2):466–70.

Chang MY, Hogan AD, Rakes GP, Ingram JM, Hoover GE, Platts-Mills TAE, Heymann PW. Salivary cotinine levels in children presenting with wheezing to an emergency department. *Pediatric Pulmonology.* 2000;29(4):257–63.

Chen Y. Environmental tobacco smoke, low birth weight, and hospitalization for respiratory disease. *American Journal of Respiratory and Critical Care Medicine.* 1994;150(1):54–8.

Chen Y, Li WX, Yu SZ, Qian WH. Chang-Ning epidemiological study of children's health. I: passive smoking and children's respiratory diseases. *International Journal of Epidemiology.* 1988a;17(2):348–55.

Chen Y, Rennie DC, Dosman JA. Influence of environmental tobacco smoke on asthma in nonallergic and allergic children. *Epidemiology.* 1996;7(5):536–9.

Christie G, Helms P. Childhood asthma: what is it and where is it going [review]? *Thorax.* 1995;50(10):1027–30.

Colley JRT. Respiratory symptoms in children and parental smoking and phlegm production. *British Medical Journal.* 1974;2(912):201–4.

Colley JRT, Holland WW, Corkhill RT. Influence of passive smoking and parental phlegm on pneumonia and bronchitis in early childhood. *Lancet.* 1974;2(7888):1031–4.

Collins MH, Moessinger AC, Kleinerman J, Bassi J, Rosso P, Collins AM, James LS, Blanc WA. Fetal lung hypoplasia associated with maternal smoking: a morphometric analysis. *Pediatric Research.* 1985;19(4):408–12.

Cook DG, Strachan DP. Health effects of passive smoking: 3. Parental smoking and prevalence of respiratory symptoms and asthma in school age children. *Thorax.* 1997;52(12):1081–94.

Cook DG, Strachan DP. Health effects of passive smoking: 7. Parental smoking, bronchial reactivity and peak flow variability in children. *Thorax.* 1998;53(4):295–301.

Cook, DG, Strachan DP. Health effects of passive smoking: 10. Summary of effects of parental smoking on the respiratory health of children and implications for research. *Thorax.* 1999;54(4):357–66.

Cook DG, Strachan DP, Carey IM. Health effects of passive smoking: 9. Parental smoking and spirometric indices in children. *Thorax.* 1998;53(10):884–93.

Cook DG, Whincup PH, Jarvis MJ, Strachan DP, Papa- costa O, Bryant A. Passive exposure to tobacco smoke in children aged 5–7: individual, family, and community factors. *British Medical Journal.* 1994;308(6925):384–9.

Dejin-Karlsson E, Hanson BS, Ostergren PO, Sjoberg NO, Marsal K. Does passive smoking in early pregnancy increase the risk of small-for-gesta tional-age infants? *American Journal of Public Health.* 1998;88(10):1523–7.

Department of Health Committee on the Medical Effects of Air Pollutants. *Asthma and Outdoor Air Pollution.* London: HMSO, 1995.

Dezateux C, Stocks J. Lung development and early ori gins of childhood respiratory illness. *British Medical Bulletin.* 1997;53(1):40–57.

DiFranza JR, Lew RA. Morbidity and mortality in chil dren associated with the use of tobacco products by other people. *Pediatrics.* 1996;97(4):560–8.

Divers WA Jr, Wilkes MM, Babaknia A, Yen SS. Mater nal smoking and elevation of catecholamines and metabolites in the amniotic fluid. *American Journal of Obstetrics and Gynecology.* 1981;141(6):625–8.

Edwards K, Braun KM, Evans G, Sureka AO, Fan S. Mainstream and sidestream cigarette smoke condensates suppress macrophage responsiveness to interferon . *Human and Experimental Toxicology.* 1999;18(4):233–40.

Egger M, Smith GD, Altman DG, editors. *Systematic Reviews in Health Care: Meta-analysis in Context.* 2nd ed. London: BMJ Publishing Group, 2001.

Elliot J, Vullermin P, Carroll N, James A, Robinson P. Increased airway smooth muscle in sudden infant death syndrome. *American Journal of Respiratory and Critical Care Medicine.* 1999;160(1):313–6.

Forsthuber T, Yip HC, Lehmann PV. Induction of TH1 and TH2 immunity in neonatal mice. *Science.* 1996;271(5256):1728–30.

Gardner G, Frank AL, Taber LH. Effects of social and family factors on viral respiratory infection and illness in the first year of life. *Journal of Epidemiology and Community Health.* 1984;38(1):42–8.

Graham NM. The epidemiology of acute respiratory infections in children and adults: a global perspec tive. *Epidemiologic Reviews.* 1990;12:149–78.

Gulya AJ. Environmental tobacco smoke and otitis media [review]. *Otolaryngology—Head and Neck Surgery.* 1994;111(1):6–8.

Halken S, Host A, Nilsson L, Taudorf E. Passive smok ing as a risk factor for development of obstructive respiratory disease and allergic sensitization. *Allergy.* 1995;50(2):97–105.

Hall CB, Hall WJ, Gala CL, MaGill FB, Leddy JP. Long-term prospective study in children after respiratory syncytial virus infection. *Journal of Pediatrics.* 1984;105(3):358–64.

Halonen M, Stern D, Lyle S, Wright A, Taussig L, Martinez FD. Relationship of total serum IgE levels in cord and 9-month sera of infants. *Clinical and Experimental Allergy.* 1991;21(2):235–41.

Hanke W, Kalinka J, Florek E, Sobala W. Passive smoking and pregnancy outcome in central Poland. *Human and Experimental Toxicology.* 1999;18(4):265–71.

Hanrahan JP, Tager IB, Segal MR, Tosteson TD, Castile RG, Van Vunakis H, Weiss ST, Speizer FE. The effect of maternal smoking during pregnancy on early infant lung function. *American Review of Respiratory Diseases.* 1992;145(5):129–35.

Harlap S, Davies AM. Infant admissions to hospital and maternal smoking. *Lancet.* 1974;1(7857):529–32.

Hasday JD, Bascom R, Costa JJ, Fitzgerald T, Dubin W. Bacterial endotoxin is an active component of cigarette smoke. *Chest.* 1999;115(3):829–35.

Hayes EB, Hurwitz ES, Schonberger LB, Anderson LJ. Respiratory syncytial virus outbreak on American Samoa: evaluation of risk factors. *American Journal of Diseases of Children.* 1989;143(3):316–21.

Hoo A-F, Henschen M, Dezateux C, Costeloe K, Stocks J. Respiratory function among preterm infants whose mothers smoked during pregnancy. *American Journal of Respiratory and Critical Care Medicine.* 1998;158(3):700–5.

Hunt LW, Gleich GJ, Ohnishi T, Weiler DA, Mansfield ES, Kita H, Sur S. Endotoxin contamination causes neutrophilia following pulmonary allergen challenge. *American Journal of Respiratory and Critical Care Medicine.* 1994;149(6):1471–5.

Ingalls RR, Heine H, Lien E, Yoshimura A, Golenbock D. Lipopolysaccharide recognition, CD14, and lipo polysaccharide receptors. *Infectious Disease Clinics of North America.* 1999;13(2):341–53, vii.

Irvine L, Crombie IK, Clark RA, Slane PW, Goodman KE, Feyerabend C, Cater JI. What determines lev els of passive smoking in children with asthma? *Thorax.* 1997;52(9):766–9.

Jin C, Rossignol AM. Effects of passive smoking on respiratory illness from birth to age eighteen months, in Shanghai, People's Republic of China. *Journal of Pediatrics.* 1993;123(4):553–8.

Jones JG, Minty BD, Lawler P, Hulands G, Crawley JC, Veall N. Increased alveolar epithelial permeability in cigarette smokers. *Lancet.* 1980;1(8159):66–8.

Kershaw CR. Passive smoking, potential atopy and asthma in the first five years. *Journal of the Royal Society of Medicine.* 1987;80(11):683–8.

Kjellman NI. Effect of parental smoking on IgE levels in children [letter]. *Lancet.* 1981;1(8227):993–4.

Klig JE, Chen L. Lower respiratory infections in chil dren. *Current Opinion in Pediatrics.* 2003;15(1):121–6.

Kraemer MJ, Richardson MA, Weiss NS, Furukawa CT, Shapiro GG, Pierson WE, Bierman CW. Risk factors for persistent middle-ear effusions: otitis media, catarrh, cigarette smoke exposure, and atopy. *Journal of the American Medical Association.* 1983;249(8):1022–5.

Lee LY, Widdicombe JG. Modulation of airway sensitivity to inhaled irritants: role of inflamma tory mediators. *Environmental Health Perspectives.* 2001;109(Suppl 4):585–9.

Lewis KW, Bosque EM. Deficient hypoxia awakening response in infants of smoking mothers: possible relationship to sudden infant death syndrome. *Journal of Pediatrics.* 1995;127(5):691–9.

Li JSM, Peat JK, Xuan W, Berry G. Meta-analysis on the association between environmental tobacco smoke (ETS) exposure and the prevalence of lower respiratory tract infection in early childhood. *Pediatric Pulmonology* 1999;27(1):5–13.

Lieberman E, Torday J, Barbieri R, Cohen A, Van Vunakis H, Weiss ST. Association of intrauter ine cigarette smoke exposure with indices of fetal lung maturation. *Obstetrics and Gynecology.* 1992;79(4):564–70.

Lodrup Carlsen KC, Jaakkola JJ, Nafstad P, Carlsen KH. In utero exposure to cigarette smoking influ ences lung function at birth. *European Respiratory Journal.* 1997;10(8):1774–9.

Magnusson CG. Maternal smoking influences cord serum IgE and IgD levels and increases the risk for subsequent infant allergy. *Journal of Allergy and Clinical Immunology.* 1986;78(5 Pt 1):898–904.

Mainous AG 3rd, Hueston WJ. Passive smoke and low birth weight: evidence of a threshold effect. *Archives of Family Medicine.* 1994;3(10):875–8.

Martinez FD, Antognoni G, Macri F, Bonci E, Midulla F, De Castro G, Ronchetti R. Parental smoking enhances bronchial responsiveness in nine-year old children. *American Review of Respiratory Diseases.* 1988;138(3):518–23.

Martinez FD, Wright AL, Taussig LM, Holberg CJ, Halonen M, Morgan WJ. Asthma and wheezing in the first six years of life: the Group Health Medi cal Associates. *New England Journal of Medicine.* 1995;332(3):133–8.

McConnochie KM, Roghmann KJ. Parental smoking, presence of older siblings, and family history of asthma increase risk of bronchiolitis. *American Journal of Diseases of Children.* 1986;140(8):806–12.

Michel O, Kips J, Duchateau J, Vertongen F, Robert L, Collet H, Pauwels R, Sergysels R. Severity of asthma is related to endotoxin in house dust. *American Journal of Respiratory and Critical Care Medicine.* 1996;154(6 Pt 1):1641–6.

Michie C. Th1 and Th2 cytokines in pregnancy, from a fetal viewpoint [letter]. *Immunology Today.* 1998;19(7):333–4.

Misra DP, Nguyen RHN. Environmental tobacco smoke and low birth weight: a hazard in the workplace? *Environmental Health Perspectives.* 1999;107(Suppl 6):879–904.

Monto AS. Epidemiology of viral respiratory infections. *American Journal of Medicine.* 2002;112(6A):4S–12S.

Murray AB, Morrison BJ. It is children with atopic dermatitis who develop asthma more frequently if the mother smokes. *Journal of Allergy and Clinical Immunology.* 1990;86(5):732–9.

Mutoh T, Bonham AC, Kott KS, Joad JP. Chronic exposure to sidestream tobacco smoke augments lung C-fiber responsiveness in young guinea pigs. *Journal of Applied Physiology.* 1999;87(2):757–68.

National Cancer Institute. *Health Effects of Exposure to Environmental Tobacco Smoke: The Report of the California Environmental Protection Agency.* Smoking and Tobacco Control Monograph No. 10. Bethesda (MD): U.S. Department of Health and Human Ser vices, National Institutes of Health, National Can cer Institute, 1999. NIH Publication No. 99-4645.

National Research Council. *Research Priorities for Airborne Particulate Matter. IV: Continuing Research Progress.* Washington: National Academies Press, 2004.

Niewoehner DE, Kleinerman J, Rice DB. Pathologic changes in the peripheral airways of young ciga rette smokers. *New England Journal of Medicine.* 1974;291(15):755–8.

Norman-Taylor W, Dickinson VA. Danger for chil dren in smoking families. *Community Medicine.* 1972;128(1):32–3.

Nuesslein TG, Beckers D, Rieger CHL. Cotinine in meconium indicates risk for early respiratory tract infections. *Human and Experimental Toxicology.* 1999;18(4):283–90.

Oryszczyn MP, Godin J, Annesi I, Hellier G, Kauff mann F. In utero exposure to parental smoking, coti nine measurements, and cord blood IgE. *Journal of Allergy and Clinical Immunology.* 1991;87(6):1169–74.

Ownby DR, Johnson CC, Peterson EL. Maternal smoking does not influence cord serum IgE or IgD concentrations. *Journal of Allergy and Clinical Immunology.* 1991;88(4):555–60.

Ownby DR, McCullough J. Passive exposure to cigarette smoke does not increase allergic sensiti zation in children. *Journal of Allergy and Clinical Immunology.* 1988;82(4):634–8.

Palmieri M, Longobardi G, Napolitano G, Simonetti DML. Parental smoking and asthma in childhood. *European Journal of Pediatrics.* 1990;149(10):738–40.

Park J-H, Gold DR, Spiegelman DL, Burge HA, Milton DK. House dust endotoxin and wheeze in the first year of life. *American Journal of Respiratory and Critical Care Medicine.* 2001;163(2):322–8.

Philipp K, Pateisky N, Endler M. Effects of smok ing on uteroplacental blood flow. *Gynecologic and Obstetric Investigation.* 1984;17(4):179–82.

Pierce RA, Nguyen NM. Prenatal nicotine expo sure and abnormal lung function. *American Journal of Respiratory Cell and Molecular Biology.* 2002;26(1):31–41.

Ronchetti R, Macri F, Ciofetta G, Indinnimeo L, Cutrera R, Bonci E, Antognoni G, Martinez FD. Increased serum IgE and increased prevalence of eosinophilia in 9-year-old children of smoking parents. *Journal of Allergy and Clinical Immunology.* 1990;86(3 Pt 1):400–7.

Rönmark E, Jönsson E, Platts-Mills T, Lundbäck B. Different pattern of risk factors for atopic and nonatopic asthma among children—report from the Obstructive Lung Disease in Northern Sweden Study. *Allergy.* 1999;54(9):926–35.

Rumold R, Jyrala M, Diaz-Sanchez D. Secondhand smoke induces allergic sensitization in mice. *Journal of Immunology.* 2001;167(8):4765–70.

Samet JM. Adverse effects of smoke exposure on the upper airway. *Tobacco Control.* 2004;13(Suppl 1): i57–i60.

Samet JM, Tager IB, Speizer FE. The relationship between respiratory illness in childhood and chronic air-flow obstruction in adulthood. *American Review of Respiratory Disease.* 1983;127(4):508–23.

Scientific Committee on Tobacco and Health. *Report of the Scientific Committee on Tobacco and Health.* Lon don: The Stationary Office, 1998.

Sekhon HS, Jia Y, Raab R, Kuryatov A, Pankow JF, Whitsett JA, Lindstrom J, Spindel ER. Prenatal nicotine increases pulmonary a7 nicotine recep tor expression and alters fetal lung develop ment in monkeys. *Journal of Clinical Investigation.* 1999;103(5):637–47.

Sekhon HS, Keller JA, Proskocil BJ, Martin EL, Spin dler ER. Maternal nicotine exposure upregulates collagen gene expression in fetal monkey lung:

associated with a7 nicotine acetylcholine receptors. *American Journal of Respiratory Cell and Molecular Biology.* 2002;26(1):10–3.

Seymour BW, Pinkerton KE, Friebertshauser KE, Coffman RL, Gershwin LJ. Second-hand smoke is an adjuvant for T helper-2 responses in a murine model of allergy. *Journal of Immunology.* 1997;159(12):6169–75.

Silverman M. Out of the mouths of babes and suck lings: lessons from early childhood asthma. *Thorax.* 1993;48(12):1200–4.

Simani AS, Inoue S, Hogg JC. Penetration of the respi ratory epithelium of guinea pigs following expo sure to cigarette smoke. *Laboratory Investigation.* 1974;31(1):75–81.

Smith KR, Samet JM, Romieu I, Bruce N. Indoor air pollution in developing countries and acute lower respiratory infections in children. *Thorax.* 2000;55(6):518–32.

Stankus RP, Menon PK, Rando RJ, Glindmeyer H, Salvaggio JE, Lehrer SB. Cigarette smoke-sensitive asthma: challenge studies. *Journal of Allergy and Clinical Immunology.* 1988;82(3 Pt 1):331–8.

Stein RT, Holberg CJ, Morgan WJ, Wright AL, Lom bardi E, Taussig L, Martinez FD. Peak flow vari ability, methacholine responsiveness and atopy as markers for detecting different wheezing pheno types in childhood. *Thorax.* 1997;52(11):946–52.

Stick SM, Burton PR, Gurrin L, Sly PD, LeSouef PN. Effects of maternal smoking during pregnancy and a family history of asthma on respiratory function in newborn infants. *Lancet.* 1996;348(9034):1060–4.

Strachan DP, Butland BK, Anderson HR. Incidence and prognosis of asthma and wheezing illness from early childhood to age 33 in a national British cohort. *British Medical Journal* 1996;312(7040):1195–9.

Strachan DP, Cook DG. Health effects of passive smoking. 1: parental smoking and lower respira tory illness in infancy and early childhood. *Thorax.* 1997;52(10):905–14.

Strachan DP, Cook DG. Health effects of passive smoking. 4: parental smoking, middle ear dis ease and adenotonsillectomy in children. *Thorax.* 1998a;53(1):50–6.

Strachan DP, Cook DG. Health effects of passive smoking. 5: parental smoking and allergic sensiti sation in children. *Thorax.* 1998b;53(2):117–23.

Strachan DP, Cook DG. Health effects of passive smok ing. 6: parental smoking and childhood asthma: longitudinal and case-control studies. *Thorax.* 1998c;53(3):204–12.

Tager IB, Hanrahan JP, Tosteson TD, Castile RG, Brown RW, Weiss ST, Speizer FE. Lung function, pre- and post-natal smoke exposure, and wheezing in the first year of life. *American Review of Respiratory Disease.* 1993;147(4):811–7.

Tager IB, Ngo L, Hanrahan JP. Maternal smoking dur ing pregnancy: effects on lung function during the first 18 months of life. *American Journal of Respiratory and Critical Care Medicine.* 1995;152(3):977–83.

Thaler I, Goodman JD, Dawes GS. Effects of mater nal cigarette smoking on fetal breathing and fetal movements. *American Journal of Obstetrics and Gynecology.* 1980;138(3):282–7.

Thornton AJ, Lee PN. Parental smoking and middle ear disease in children: a review of the evidence. *Indoor and Built Environment.* 1999;8(1):21–39.

Tuli MK, Wale JL, Holt PG, Sly PD. Modification of the inflammatory response to allergen challenge after exposure to bacterial lipopolysaccharide. *American Journal of Respiratory Cell and Molecular Biology.* 2000;22(5):604–12.

Uhari M, Mäntysaari K, Niemelä M. A meta-analytic review of the risk factors for acute otitis media. *Clinical Infectious Diseases.* 1996;22(6):1079–83.

U.S. Department of Health and Human Services. *The Health Consequences of Smoking: Chronic Obstructive Lung Disease. A Report of the Surgeon General.* Rock ville (MD): U.S. Department of Health and Human Services, Public Health Service, Office on Smoking and Health, 1984. DHHS Publication No. (PHS) 84-50205.

U.S. Department of Health and Human Services. *The Health Consequences of Involuntary Smoking. A Report of the Surgeon General.* Rockville (MD): U.S. Department of Health and Human Services, Public Health Service, Centers for Disease Control, Center for Health Promotion and Education, Office on Smoking and Health, 1986. DHHS Publication No. (CDC) 87-8398.

U.S. Department of Health and Human Services. *Women and Smoking. A Report of the Surgeon General.* Rockville (MD): U.S. Department of Health and Human Services, Public Health Service, Office of the Surgeon General, 2001.

U.S. Department of Health and Human Services. *The Health Consequences of Smoking: A Report of the Surgeon General.* Atlanta: U.S. Department of Health and Human Services, Centers for Disease Control and Prevention, National Center for Chronic Dis ease Prevention and Health Promotion, Office on Smoking and Health, 2004.

Victora CG, Fuchs SC, Flores JAC, Fonseca W, Kirk wood B. Risk factors for pneumonia among chil dren in a Brazilian metropolitan area. *Pediatrics.* 1994;93(6 Pt 1):977–85.

Vidic B. Transplacental effect of environmental pol lutants on interstitial composition and diffusion capacity for exchange of gases of pulmonary paren chyma in neonatal rat. *Bulletin de l'Association des Anatomistes. (Nancy)* 1991;75(229):153–5.

Weiss ST, Tager IB, Munoz A, Speizer FE. The rela tionship of respiratory infections in early childhood to the occurrence of increased levels of bronchial responsiveness and atopy. *American Review of Respiratory Diseases.* 1985;131(4):573–8.

Wilson NM. Wheezy bronchitis revisited. *Archives of Disease in Childhood.* 1989;64(8):1194–9.

Wilson NM. The significance of early wheezing. *Clinical and Experimental Allergy.* 1994;24(6):522–9.

World Health Organization. *International Consultation on Environmental Tobacco Smoke. (ETS) and Child Health: Consultation Report.* Geneva: World Health Organization, Tobacco Free Initiative, 1999. Report No. WHO/NCD/TFI/99.10.

Young S, Sherrill DL, Arnott J, Diepeveen D, LeSouëf PN, Landau LI. Parental factors affecting respira tory function during the first year of life. *Pediatric Pulmonology.* 2000b;29(5):331–40.

In: Children and Secondhand Smoke Exposure ISBN: 978-1-60692-587-4
Editor: J. R. Harrington © 2009 Nova Science Publishers, Inc.

Chapter 5

EXCERPTS FROM CHAPTER 10. CONTROL OF SECONDHAND SMOKE EXPOSURE

INTRODUCTION

This chapter examines measures to control exposure to secondhand smoke in public places, workplaces, and homes, including legislation, education, and approaches based on building designs and operations. The discussion reviews progress toward smoke- free indoor spaces in the United States during the past three decades, including approaches that have been employed to reduce exposure, in the context of exten sive scientific evidence on health effects and control measures. Table 10.1 provides a chronology of some landmark or exemplary efforts at all levels of government to limit exposure to secondhand smoke.

ATTITUDES AND BELIEFS ABOUT SECONDHAND SMOKE

A number of nationally representative stud ies that assessed public attitudes toward smoking in public places have been published since the 1960s. The 1989 report of the Surgeon General considered studies from the previous three decades (USDHHS 1989). The most recent studies are the NCI's Tobacco Use Supplement to the Current Population Survey (CPS) (USDOC 1985, 2004) and the National Health Interview Survey (NHIS) (National Center for Health Statistics [NCHS] 2004). CPS is a monthly survey of about 50,000 households. Questions on smoking were included in September 1992, January

1993, and May 1993 (Gerlach et al. 1997), and the questions were repeated during the same months in 1995–1996, 1998–1999, and 2001–2002 (Shopland et al. 2001; CDC, NCHS, NHIS, public use data tapes, 2001–2002). In the text that follows, the dates of surveys are referred to as 1993, 1996, 1999, and 2002, respectively. The NHIS is a multipurpose health survey conducted by CDC. Because the CPS and NHIS represent the most recent data available using nationally representative sam ples, this Surgeon General's report includes extensive analyses of these data.

Trends in Beliefs About Health Risks of Secondhand Smoke

Surveys conducted in recent years consistently show that substantial majorities of the U.S. public believe that secondhand smoke exposure is a health hazard for nonsmokers. In both 1992 and 2000, NHIS asked respondents if they agreed with the statement that secondhand smoke is harmful. In both years, more than 80 percent of respondents agreed. Individ uals with more years of education were more likely to believe that secondhand smoke is harmful. According to data from the 2001 annual Social Climate Survey of Tobacco Control, 95 percent of the adults agreed that parental secondhand smoke was harmful to children, and 96 percent considered tobacco company claims that secondhand smoke is not harmful to be untruth ful (McMillen et al. 2003).

POLICY APPROACHES

During the past 30 years, policies to restrict smoking in public places and in workplaces have been implemented with increasing success. Over time, the number, strength, and coverage of these policies have steadily increased. Although not subject to regulation, exposure in the home (the main source of exposure for most children at present) has also been the focus of intervention research designed, to the extent pos sible, to help smoking parents protect their children from secondhand smoke exposure and to help smok ers protect nonsmoking spouses and other adult non smokers who live with them.

Household Smoking Rules

Home smoking restrictions are private house hold rules that are adopted voluntarily by household members. They can include comprehensive rules that make homes smokefree in all areas at all times and less comprehensive rules that restrict smoking to cer tain places or times (e.g., allowing smoking only in specific rooms, designating certain rooms as smoke- free, allowing smoking only when no children are present, etc.) (Pyle et al. 2005). The only approach that effectively protects nonsmokers from secondhand smoke exposure is a rule making the home completely smoke-free (Levy et al. 2004).

Smoke-free home rules and other home smok ing restrictions may be implemented for a variety of reasons, including

- to protect children in the household from secondhand smoke exposure;
- to protect pregnant women in the household from secondhand smoke exposure;
- to protect nonsmoking spouses or other nonsmoking adult household members from secondhand smoke exposure;
- to protect children or adults who have health conditions that are exacerbated by secondhand smoke exposure or who are at risk for health conditions that can be triggered by secondhand smoke (e.g., a child with asthma, an adult with or at special risk for heart disease);
- to help smokers in the household cut down their cigarette consumption;
- to help smokers quit;
- to help smokers who have quit maintain abstinence;
- to set a positive example for children and youth in the household, to prevent them from becoming smokers themselves;
- aesthetic, hygienic, economic, and safety con siderations, including eliminating the odor of secondhand smoke, eliminating cigarette burns, and eliminating the risk of fires caused by discarded cigarettes; and
- simply because no one in the household smokes anymore (Ferrence et al. 2005).

Prevalence and Correlates

Reducing secondhand smoke exposure in the home is important because the home is a major source of exposure for children and for those nonsmok ing adults who are not exposed elsewhere. Reduc ing exposure in this setting is challenging, however, because there are no clearly established interventions that effectively reduce exposure at home. In addition, because smoke-free home rules are adopted voluntarily, rather than imposed by government bodies or employers, the prevalence of these rules is an important indicator of changes in norms regarding the social acceptability of smoking. In the text that follows, the definition of "children" varies across the studies cited.

In the past decade, substantial increases have occurred in the number of U.S. households with private rules to limit secondhand smoke exposure within the home. Even smokers are increasingly adopting such rules. One of the best data sources available on children's secondhand smoke exposure in the home is the NHIS. This information can be derived from NHIS data by correlating data on smoking in the home with data on households with children. NHIS data show that the proportion of children aged 6 years and younger who are regularly exposed to secondhand smoke in their homes fell from 27 percent in 1994 to 20 percent in 1998. A recent study by Soliman and colleagues (2004) examined data from the NHIS and found that the prevalence of secondhand smoke exposure in homes with children fell from 35.6 percent in 1992 to 25.1 percent in 2000. The prevalence of adult smoking fell by a smaller amount during this same period, from 26.5 to 23.3 percent, indicating that a portion of the reduced exposure can be explained by the increase in home smoking rules. Home exposures declined across all racial, ethnic, educational, and income groups that were analyzed. Farkas and colleagues (2000) analyzed data from adolescents aged 15 through 17 years from the 1993 and 1996 CPS. Of those respondents, 48 percent lived in smoke-free households in 1993 and 55 percent lived in smoke-free homes by 1996.

The CPS data show that the percentage of smoke-free homes increased by 40 percent between 1993 and 2002, from 43 to 66 percent. Households with a smoker in the home had lower rates of smoke-free home rules than did households without a smoker; however, the prevalence of smoke-free rules in homes with smokers increased by 110 percent between 1993 and 1999. In a 1997 survey in Oregon, Pizacani and colleagues (2003) found similar differences in the prevalence of smoke-free home rules between nonsmoking households (85 percent) and households with one or more smokers (38 percent). These trends of smoke-free home rules were observed in all four regions of the country in the CPS data. Individuals living in the West reported higher rates of smoke-free homes, but the largest increases between 1993 and 2002 were in the South and the Midwest. Similarly, there were wide variations among states in the percentage of individuals reporting household smoking bans. Utah reported the highest rate (83 percent), followed by California (78 percent), Arizona (76 percent), and Idaho (74 per cent).

The presence of a child younger than 13 years of age was associated with only a slight increase in the rate of smoke-free homes compared with homes where there were no children under 13 years of age. However, a survey of 598 adult smokers living in an inner-city neighborhood in Kansas City (Missouri) found that after adjusting for age, race, gender, and education, a rule banning smoking or restricting it to designated locations in the home was significantly more likely in households with a child (OR = 2.63 [95 percent CI, 1.70–4.08]) or a nonsmoking adult part ner (OR = 2.07 [95 percent CI, 1.19–3.61]) (Okah et al. 2002).

Households with lower incomes reported lower rates of smoke-free home rules compared with higher income households. The amount smoked was higher in lower income homes, whether or not a smoker resided in the home (Okah et al. 2002).

EPA conducted a national telephone survey in 2003 on children's secondhand smoke exposure and childhood asthma among a random digit-dialed sam ple of U.S. households, involving 14,685 interviews (USEPA 2005). The survey yielded the following results:

- Approximately 11 percent of children aged six years and under were reported to be exposed to secondhand smoke on a regular basis (four or more days per week) in their home.
- Secondhand smoke exposure is significantly higher in households at and below the poverty level.
- Parents account for the vast majority of exposure in homes (almost 90 percent of the exposure), followed by grandparents and other relatives living in the home.
- The presence of a child with asthma in the home was not associated with reduced exposure, even in homes with younger children. Children with asthma were just as likely to be exposed to secondhand smoke as children in general.
- The contribution of visitors to the regular expo sure of children to secondhand smoke was neg ligible. In households with children aged 6 years or younger, only 0.3 percent of children were exposed to secondhand smoke by visitors alone. Similarly, only 0.5 percent of children under 18 were exposed solely by visitors.

The prevalence of smoke-free household rules has been studied in California, which has undertaken a campaign to promote smoke-free homes as part of its comprehensive statewide tobacco control program (Gilpin et al. 2001). The 1999 California Tobacco Sur vey found that 73.2 percent of California homes had a smoke-free rule in place. This finding represented an increase of 30 percent from 1993. In addition, nearly half (47.2 percent) of the smokers lived in a smoke- free home—an increase of 135 percent from 1993. An additional 21.8 percent of smokers lived in homes with some smoking restrictions. Consistent with these increases, the percentage of children and adolescents protected from secondhand smoke exposure at home increased by 15 percent during that same time period to 88.6 percent (Gilpin et al. 2001).

Gilpin and colleagues (1999) used data from the 1996 California Tobacco Survey (n = 8,904) to evalu¬ ate factors associated with the adoption of smoke-free home rules. The data showed that male smokers were more likely than female smokers to report smoke- free homes, and household smoking bans were less likely with the increased age of current smokers in the household. Hispanic and Asian smokers were more likely to report smoke-free homes (58 percent and 43 percent, respectively) than were non-Hispanic Whites (32 percent); African Americans were the least likely to report smoke-free homes (23 percent). Living in a household with a child or with nonsmoking adults predicted a smoke-free household. After adjusting for demographics, the investigators noted that smokers were nearly six times more likely to report living in a smoke-free home if they lived with a nonsmoking adult and child compared with smokers who lived in homes without children or adult nonsmokers (59 per cent versus 15 percent, respectively).

Effect of Household Smoking Rules on Secondhand Smoke Exposure

During the past two decades, several data sources have consistently shown that a large proportion of children in the United States were regularly exposed to secondhand smoke. For example, 1988 NHIS data revealed that 42.4 percent of children aged five years and younger lived with at least one smoker (Over peck and Moss 1991). Data from the 1991 NHIS indi cated that 31.2 percent of children aged 10 years and younger were exposed daily to secondhand smoke in their homes (Mannino et al. 1996). An important find ing was that children from lower income families were significantly more likely to be exposed to secondhand smoke than were children from higher income fami lies. For example, 41 percent of children from lower income families were exposed daily compared with only 21 percent of children from higher income families. CDC's 2005 Third National Report on Human Exposure to Environmental Chemicals, drawing on data from NHANES, reported that median cotinine levels measured during 1999–2002 have fallen by 68 percent among children, by 69 percent among adolescents, and by 75 percent among adults when compared with median levels from 1988–1991. However, the data also show that children's cotinine levels are twice as high as those of adults (CDC 2005b).

In an intervention study of low-income households with at least one child under three years of age, the median household nicotine concentration was 3.3 $\mu g/m^3$ (Emmons et al. 2001). A recent study that measured cotinine levels in infants and nicotine levels in household dust, in the air, and on household surfaces found that smoke-free home rules may substantially reduce, but may not completely eliminate, household contamination from secondhand smoke, including secondhand smoke exposure of infants (Matt et al. 2004). The study found that infants living with smokers in homes with smoke-free rules had lower cotinine levels compared with infants from homes with smokers without such rules, but cotinine levels were higher compared with infants from homes without smokers. The same was true of nicotine levels in household dust, in air, and on household surfaces. One possible explanation for this finding is that even with smoke-free home rules, secondhand smoke may enter the house in the air, on dust, or on the smoker's breath or clothing. And there is always the possibility that some smokers may not be consistently complying with the rules or may be overstating the rules. Exposure does not appear to be lower in homes with children who are at particular risk from secondhand smoke, such as children with asthma. Kane and colleagues (1999) conducted home visits of 828 households in a lower income section of Buffalo (New York) to identify 167 persons of all ages with asthma and 161 persons without asthma. Self-reported household secondhand smoke exposure levels were similar in both groups— half of the households reported exposure.

Interventions to Reduce Home-Based Secondhand Smoke Exposure of Children

Because secondhand smoke exposure poses serious health risks to children and because the home is the major source of exposure for children, a number of public health practitioners, tobacco control programs, and other organizations at the local, state, and national levels have carried out activities intended to reduce children's secondhand smoke exposure in the home. As the lead federal government agency in this area, EPA has played an especially significant role at the national level. EPA has collaborated with the health care community, state and local tobacco control programs, and other organizations to mar shal efforts to institutionalize smoke-free home rules (USDHHS 2003). The American Legacy Foundation also launched a media initiative in 2005 to promote smoke-free homes and vehicles (American Legacy Foundation 2005).

However, few interventions to reduce children's secondhand smoke exposure have been systemati cally evaluated. *The Guide to Community Preventive Services* found insufficient evidence for the effective ness of community educational initiatives designed to reduce secondhand smoke exposure in the home (Task Force on Community Preventive Services 2005). In a systematic review, the Guide was able to identify only three relevant studies and only one study that met its criteria.

Table 10.16 summarizes a number of relevant studies (see page 622 in the full report). The early studies did not show a significant effect on objective exposure measures, although some showed reduc tions of self-reported exposure.

Two trials in the United States found substan tial reductions in secondhand smoke exposure among healthy children as a result of an intervention (Hovell et al. 2000a; Emmons et al. 2001). In a randomized controlled trial of 291 smoking parents of young chil dren, Emmons and colleagues (2001) used a motiva tional intervention to reduce household secondhand smoke exposure. Participants were low-income fami lies, recruited through primary care settings, with children younger than three years of age. Participants were randomly assigned to either the motivational intervention group or a self-help comparison group; follow-up assessments were conducted at three months and six months. The motivational intervention con sisted of one 30- to 45-minute motivational interview session at the participant's home with a trained health educator and four follow-up telephone counseling calls. The intervention included feedback to partici pants regarding baseline levels of airborne nicotine and CO in their homes. Families in the self-help group were mailed a copy of a smoking cessation manual, a secondhand smoke reduction tip sheet, and a resource guide. Household nicotine levels were measured by a passive diffusion monitor. The six-month nicotine levels were significantly lower in motivational inter vention households than in the self-help households. Repeated measures of analysis of variance across baseline, three-month, and six-month time points showed a significant time-by-treatment interaction— indicating that patterns over time differ by treatment group— whereby nicotine levels for the motivational intervention group decreased significantly, and nico tine levels for the self-help group increased but were not significantly different from baseline.

Hovell and colleagues (2000a) evaluated a seven-session, three-month counseling intervention with a randomized trial design involving 108 moth ers who had a child under four years of age. Reported exposure of children declined from 27.3 cigarettes per week at baseline to 4.5 cigarettes per week at 3 months and to 3.7 cigarettes per week at 12 months in the counseled group. The investigators also observed reductions in exposure among the controls, but the reductions among the intervention participants were significantly greater. At the 12-month follow-up comparison between the intervention group and the controls, the level of self-reported exposure in the intervention group was 41.2 percent of the exposure of the controls from maternal smoking and 46 percent of the exposure of the controls from all sources com bined (Hovell et al. 2000a). Urinary cotinine concen trations among children decreased by 4 percent in the intervention group but increased by 85 percent in the control group.

Other studies have evaluated family interven tions designed to reduce secondhand smoke exposure among children with asthma. Hovell and colleagues (2002) demonstrated a significant impact on self- reported exposure among a general population of families with children who have asthma and an impact on self-reported exposure and cotinine levels among Hispanic families.

Gehrman and Hovell (2003) reviewed 19 studies of interventions to reduce secondhand smoke expo sure among children in the home setting that were pub lished between 1987 and 2002. The interventions fell into two categories: (1) physician-based interventions, which consisted of information and recommenda tions delivered orally by a physician or nurse during a regularly scheduled appointment (e.g., a well-baby or immunization visit) in a pediatrician's office or other health care facility, and (2) home-based interventions, which consisted of counseling delivered by a nurse or a trained research assistant during a home visit. The main outcome of interest was children's secondhand smoke exposure, with parental smoking cessation as a secondary outcome of interest in some studies. Children's exposure was primarily measured through parental self-report, with some studies also measuring children's urinary cotinine levels. Of the 19 studies, 11 reported significant reductions in secondhand smoke exposure. However, only one of the eight studies that monitored children's cotinine levels reported signifi cant differences in cotinine levels between treatment and control groups. Effect sizes (measured as Cohen's d) ranged from -0.14 to 1.04, with a mean effect size of 0.34. The review suggests that interventions in this area can achieve at least small to moderate effects.

Gehrman and Hovell (2003) concluded that home-based interventions, which tended to be more intensive in terms of frequency and duration of con tact, generally appeared to be more effective than physician-based interventions, which tended to be less intensive. Seven of the eight exclusively home-based interventions assessed yielded significant effects, compared with 4 of the 10 physician-based interventions. The review also found that interventions that were explicitly based on behavior change theory (e.g., behavior modification theory, social learning/cognitive theory) appeared to be more likely to be effective, with eight of the nine interventions that fell into this category registering significant secondhand smoke reductions.

Gehrman and Hovell (2003) suggest that optimal interventions should combine physician- and home- based approaches, combine immediate steps to reduce children's secondhand smoke exposure with cessation support for parents who want to quit, be based on behavior change theory (especially in terms of providing participants with concrete skills and strategies to help them achieve the desired outcomes), foster participants' self-efficacy and provide them with ongoing reinforcement for positive behavior changes, and be sustained over time. The study also suggests that future studies should explore approaches to increasing the effectiveness of physician-based interventions, for example, equipping mothers with skills to deal with spouses or other household members who are contributing to children's secondhand smoke exposure. In addition, studies should examine efficacy of other interventions, including group interventions (as opposed to one-on-one interventions), the use of motivational interviewing, exploring the link between reducing children's secondhand smoke exposure and increasing parental cessation, and interventions directed at children (as opposed to interventions directed at parents). The authors also emphasize the importance of evaluating interventions; they note, for example, that while "home-based interventions may be particularly promising, . . .future research should be done in a systematic, replicable manner so that investigators can make more direct comparisons" (Gehrman and Hovell 2003, p. 297). Finally, in addition to refining interventions directed at individual behavior change, efforts should be continued to increase public awareness and smoking restrictions.

Hovell and colleagues (2000b) examined the effectiveness of available approaches to reducing secondhand smoke exposure among children. The study identified three trials reporting that repeated counseling reduced quantitative measures of secondhand smoke exposure in asthmatic children and one controlled trial reporting that repeated physician counseling directed toward reducing secondhand smoke exposure increased parental cessation. Controlled trials of clinicians' one-time counseling yielded null results. The study concluded that one-time clinical interventions appeared marginally effective or ineffective. Repeated minimal interventions, while not consistently yielding changes in secondhand smoke exposure, appeared to hold more promise. However, the study calls for further evaluations of this approach, specifically large-scale controlled trials.

Hovell and colleagues (2000b) also note that even the interventions that appeared to reduce secondhand smoke exposure rarely eliminated it completely and suggest that these interventions may need to be sustained over long periods of time. The study points to a need for further research on approaches that combine counseling to reduce children's secondhand smoke exposure with subsequent counseling to help parents quit smoking. Such counseling might include interventions to address situations where the mother, who typically is the patient receiving the counseling, is not the only smoker in the household or is not a smoker at all. Other interventions might be directed at children instead of parents. Still others might address the social disparities implicit in the increased prevalence of smoking and secondhand smoke exposure among low-SES populations and some racial/ethnic groups.

Hovell and colleagues (2000b) also examined a number of other strategies for reducing children's secondhand smoke exposure, including regulatory, policy, legal, and media approaches. The study concludes by noting the importance of pursuing interventions in this area within the context of a comprehensive approach to tobacco control.

In addition to the role of the health care sector in establishing smoke-free policies and changing norms related to smoking in health care settings, the role that pediatricians can play in reducing exposure of children to secondhand smoke has drawn increasing attention. The American Academy of Pediatrics has recommended that secondhand smoke exposure of children should be discussed as part of pediatric care, and providers should follow the Agency for Healthcare Research and Quality (formerly the Agency for Health Care Policy and Research) guidelines for working with parents to quit or reduce their smoking (Etzel and Balk 1999). The American Academy of Pediatrics has identified secondhand smoke exposure as a priority area and is collaborating with EPA and others to reduce childhood exposures.

Effect on Smoking Behavior

National data have confirmed findings from California that relate household smoking rules and workplace smoking policies to smoking status. Farkas and colleagues (1999) analyzed 1993 CPS data and found that, compared with smokers living under no household smoking restrictions, smokers living under a total household smoking ban were almost four times more likely to report an attempt to quit smoking during the previous 12 months compared with smokers with no household smoking restrictions (OR = 3.86 [95 percent CI, 3.57–4.18]). Smokers who lived in a home with a partial smoking ban were almost twice as likely to report an attempt to quit during the previous 12 months (OR = 1.83 [95 percent CI, 1.72–1.92]). The investigators also noted a weaker relationship between workplace smoking bans compared with workplaces with no restrictions or restrictions less than a ban on smoking in work areas, and reporting an attempt to quit (OR = 1.14 [95 percent CI, 1.05–1.24]). Among smokers who attempted to quit in the previous year, smokers who lived under a household smoking ban had an OR of 1.65 (95 percent CI, 1.43–1.91) of abstaining for at least six months compared with smokers with no household smoking restrictions, while smokers who lived under a partial household smoking ban had an OR of 1.20 (95 percent CI, 1.05–1.38). Smokers with a workplace smoking ban who tried to quit had an OR of 1.21 (95 percent CI, 1.00–1.45) for abstaining for at least six months compared with smokers working under no workplace restrictions or some form of restriction less than a work area ban (Farkas et al. 1999).

In a recent prospective study of a population-based cohort of smokers identified from a previous telephone survey, Pizacani and colleagues (2004) found that smokers living under a full household smoking ban at baseline were twice as likely as smokers living with no ban or with a partial ban to attempt to quit and to abstain for at least one day over follow-up of about two years. The study also found that among smokers who were preparing to quit at baseline, a full ban was associated with a lower relapse rate and with more than four times the odds of abstaining for seven or more days at follow-up. These associations were not found among smokers in the precontemplation/contemplation stage of quitting. The authors concluded that full household smoking bans may facilitate cessation among smokers who are preparing to quit by increasing cessation attempts and may prolong the time to relapse among these smokers (Pizacani et al. 2004).

Important relationships have also been found between household and workplace smoking restrictions and smoking trends among adolescents. After adjusting for demographics, school enrollment, and having other smokers in the home, adolescents from smoke-free households were 26 percent less likely to be smokers than adolescents who lived in homes without smoking restrictions. Adolescents who worked indoors in smoke-free workplaces were 32 percent less likely to be smokers than adolescents whose indoor workplaces had a partial work area ban. Smoke-free home rules also increased the chances of quitting among adolescent smokers; respondents were 1.80 times more likely to be former smokers if they lived in smoke-free homes (Farkas et al. 2000). The findings of the surveys need to be interpreted with consideration of the diffi culty in inferring causal directions from cross-sectional data. The cohort study of Pizacani and colleagues (2004) would not be subject to this potential limitation.

Smoking Restrictions in Other Settings

Day Care

Day care settings present a potentially impor tant source of secondhand smoke exposure for young children. In 1995, 75 percent of children (14.4 million) younger than five years of age were in some form of regular child care arrangement (Smith 1995). A national survey conducted in 1990 of 2,003 directors of licensed day care centers found that 99 percent of these facilities were in compliance with their state laws on smoking: 55 percent of the centers were smoke- free indoors and outdoors, 26 percent were smoke- free indoors only, and 18 percent allowed restricted indoor smoking. The best predictors of more stringent employee smoking policies were locations in the West or South, smaller size, and independent ownership (Nelson et al. 1993). This survey also found that of the 40 states that regulated employee smoking in day care facilities, only 3 states banned indoor smoking (Nelson et al. 1993). In a 2004 analysis by the Ameri can Lung Association (ALA) of state laws restricting smoking, researchers identified 44 states that regu lated smoking in day care centers, of which 31 prohib ited smoking, 5 allowed smoking only in enclosed and separately ventilated areas, and 8 had some other type of restriction (ALA 2004). These results only apply to licensed facilities and not necessarily to family day care or more informal arrangements, which may be less restrictive. A large proportion of children are in nonfederally funded settings; 50 percent of children in day care are cared for by a relative in an informal setting. The smoking rules in these settings have not been studied.

In 1994, the U.S. Congress passed the *Pro- Children Act of 1994*, which prohibits smoking in Head Start facilities and in kindergarten, elementary, and secondary schools that receive federal funding from the U.S. Department of Education, the U.S. Depart ment of Agriculture, or the U.S. DHHS, with the exception of funding from Medicare or Medicaid. This legislation also applies to facilities that receive federal funding to provide children with routine health care, day care, or early childhood development services. This measure was reauthorized under the *No Child Left Behind Act of 2001*. No nationally representative survey of day care facilities has been conducted since the enactment of the *Pro-Children Act of 1994*.

Schools

During the past decade, schools have increas ingly adopted smoke-free policies to minimize pro- smoking social norms, to reduce smoking initiation rates, and to protect children from secondhand smoke exposure in the school setting.

At the federal level, the *Pro-Children Act of 1994* prohibits smoking in facilities where federally funded educational, health, library, day care, or child develop ment services are provided to children aged younger than 18 years (Federal Register 1994). The *Pro-Children Act of 1994* was reauthorized under the *No Child Left Behind Act of 2001.*

Expanding upon the *Pro-Children Act of 1994*, the CDC Guidelines for School Health Programs to Prevent Tobacco Use and Addiction recommend a tobacco-free school policy that prohibits students, staff, and visitors from using tobacco products in school buildings, on school grounds, in school vehi cles, and at school-sponsored events (including events held on and off school property) (CDC 1994). Accord ing to the guidelines, this policy should be in effect at all times, even when schools are out of session. The tobacco-free environment established by this policy protects children from secondhand smoke in school buildings and other areas that they frequent as part of their daily school experience and in particular elimi nates exposure of children with asthma to secondhand smoke (CDC 2005a). These policies also reduce chil dren's opportunities to use tobacco products and to witness others doing so, thus reinforcing the messages that children receive in school about the importance of healthy, tobacco-free lifestyles. Finally, tobacco-free school policies create young people who are prepared to—and in fact expect to—matriculate to smoke-free workplaces and communities (CDC 1994).

According to CDC's School Health Policies and Programs Study (SHPPS) 2000, 44.6 percent of schools reported tobacco-free school policies consistent with CDC recommendations, up from 36 percent in SHPPS 1994 (*Journal of School Health* 2001). The study also found that 45.5 percent of districts and 13 states reported such policies. Since 2000, the numbers of schools, districts, and states with tobacco-free school policies have continued to increase. Oregon is the most recent state to adopt such a policy. A *Healthy People 2010* objective calls for establishing comprehen sive tobacco-free policies in all junior high schools, middle schools, and senior high schools (USDHHS 2000). While substantial progress has been made on this objective, the target is not likely to be met by 2010 unless activity increases.

CONCLUSIONS

The following conclusions are supported by text in the full report that may not be included in this excerpt. The full report can be accessed at http://www.surgeongeneral.gov/library/second handsmoke/report/.

1. Workplace smoking restrictions are effective in reducing secondhand smoke exposure.
2. Workplace smoking restrictions lead to less smoking among covered workers.
3. Establishing smoke-free workplaces is the only effective way to ensure that secondhand smoke exposure does not occur in the workplace.
4. The majority of workers in the United States are now covered by smoke-free policies.
5. The extent to which workplaces are covered by smoke-free policies varies among worker groups, across states, and by sociodemographic factors. Workplaces related to the entertainment and hospitality industries have notably high potential for secondhand smoke exposure.
6. Evidence from peer-reviewed studies shows that smoke-free policies and regulations do not have an adverse economic impact on the hospitality industry.
7. Evidence suggests that exposure to secondhand smoke varies by ethnicity and gender.
8. In the United States, the home is now becoming the predominant location for exposure of children and adults to secondhand smoke.
9. Total bans on indoor smoking in hospitals, restaurants, bars, and offices substantially reduce secondhand smoke exposure, up to several orders of magnitude with incomplete compliance, and with full compliance, exposures are eliminated.
10. Exposures of nonsmokers to secondhand smoke cannot be controlled by air cleaning or mechanical air exchange.

OVERALL IMPLICATIONS

Total bans on indoor smoking in hospitals, res taurants, bars, and offices will substantially reduce secondhand smoke exposure, up to several orders of magnitude with incomplete compliance, and, with full compliance, exposures will be eliminated. Absent a ban, attempts to control secondhand smoke exposure of nonsmoking occupants or patrons have mixed results. Uncontrolled air currents, mixed return air and ventilation air, and the lack of complete physical barriers lead to persistence of some secondhand smoke exposure with partial restriction strategies. The few studies that claim unrestricted smoking in offices meets ASHRAE standards do not provide convincing evidence that exposures of nonsmokers to secondhand smoke were adequately reduced (ASHRAE 1999). Specially designed smoking areas inside a building can effectively isolate secondhand smoke, but effectiveness depends on engineering design and on high volume exhaust separated from the main AHU to maintain a negative pressure within the physically isolated area. Mechanical air cleaning has not been sufficiently effective to permit exhaust air, transported or leaked air from a designated smoking area, or air from a physically separated smoking room or lounge to be remixed with ventilation air.

Ventilation rates substantially higher than the minimums recommended by ASHRAE (1999) might dilute some secondhand smoke constituents in some indoor settings to levels indistinguishable (statistically) from levels in buildings that restrict smoking. Perhaps, under such circumstances, indoor air quality might be perceived as acceptable at the 80 per cent threshold criterion set by ASHRAE for persons voluntarily electing to be indoors in the presence of active smokers. However, this threshold criterion does not adequately account for possible health effects associated with exposure to secondhand smoke constituents even at low levels. Absent being able to specify acceptable levels of airborne contaminants and risks associated with secondhand smoke, concentration-based guidelines for secondhand smoke cannot be developed. Thus, exposure to secondhand smoke components cannot be controlled sufficiently through dilution ventilation or by typical air cleaning strategies if the goal is to achieve no risk or a negligible risk. The only effective controls that eliminate exposures of nonsmokers are the complete physical isolation of smoking areas with separate air exhausts or a total smoking ban within the structure. This conclusion echoes prior conclusions of federal agencies (USDHHS 1986; USEPA 1992; NIOSH 1991).

Despite wider adoption of smoking restrictions, exposures to secondhand smoke persist. Among adults, data from the 1991 NHIS Health Promotion and Disease Prevention Supplement indicate that 20.2 percent of lifetime nonsmokers and 23.1 percent of former smokers reported any exposure to secondhand smoke at home or at work (Mannino et al. 1997). Self-reported data from NHANES III (1988–1991) suggest that 37 percent of lifetime nonsmokers were exposed to secondhand smoke, and men (46 percent) were more likely than women (32 percent) to experience exposure (Steenland et al. 1998). Most nonsmokers were exposed in the workplace (20 percent) compared with those exposed at home (11 percent) or at both work and home (6 percent). However, Pirkle and colleagues (1996) used high-performance liquid chromatography atmospheric-pressure chemical ionization tandem mass spectrometry to analyze serum cotinine levels and found that 87 percent of nonsmokers had detectable levels. These investigators also noted that children, non-Hispanic Blacks, and males had higher levels than the rest of the populations that were studied (Pirkle et al. 1996).

Some evidence suggests that exposure among certain ethnic and gender groups may be higher. For example, Pletsch (1994) examined self-reported secondhand smoke exposure data from 4,256 Hispanic females aged 12 through 49 years who participated in the Hispanic Health and Nutrition Examination Survey (NCHS 1985). Pletsch (1994) found that 62 percent of Mexican American women, 59 percent of Puerto Rican women, and 52 percent of Cuban American women were regularly exposed to secondhand smoke at home, and 35 percent of Mexican American women, 28 percent of Puerto Rican women, and 49 percent of Cuban American women were regularly exposed at work.

According to NHIS data, most of the U.S. working population (76.5 percent) does not smoke (NCHS, public use data tape, 2002). In 2002, there were an estimated 100.3 million nonsmoking workers in the United States. In a study that compared exposure levels with OSHA's significant risk standards, more than 95 percent of the office workers exposed to secondhand smoke in the United States exceeded OSHA's significant risk level for heart disease mortality, and 60 percent exceeded the significant risk level for lung cancer mortality (Repace et al. 1998). Repace and colleagues (1998) estimated excesses of 4,000 heart disease deaths and 400 lung cancer deaths were attributable to workplace exposure.

On the basis of this review, it is clear that banning smoking from the workplace is the only effective way to ensure that exposures are not occurring. Despite reductions in workplace smoking, significant worker safety issues remain that only smoking bans can address. The home remains the most serious venue for secondhand smoke exposure.

REFERENCES

American Legacy Foundation. More than 13 million American children regularly breathing secondhand smoke in their homes, cars: American legacy Foundation and the Ad Council launch first campaign to call attention to and educate public about dangers of secondhand smoke [press release]. Washington: American Legacy Foundation, January 11, 2005.

American Lung Association. *State Legislated Actions on Tobacco Issues*. 16th Edition, 2004. Washington: American Lung Association, 2005.

American Society of Heating, Refrigerating and Air- Conditioning Engineers. ANSI/ASHRAE Standard 62-1999: Ventilation for Acceptable Indoor Air Quality. Atlanta: *American Society of Heating, Refrigerating and Air-Conditioning Engineers,* 1999.

Centers for Disease Control and Prevention. Guide lines for school health programs to prevent tobacco use and addiction. *Morbidity and Mortality Weekly Report.* 1994;43(RR-2):1–18.

Centers for Disease Control and Prevention. *Strategies for Addressing Asthma Within a Coordinated School Health Program, With Updated Resources.* Atlanta: Centers for Disease Control and Prevention, National Center for Chronic Disease Prevention and Health Promotion, 2005a.

Centers for Disease Control and Prevention. *Third National Report on Human Exposure to Environmental Chemicals.* Atlanta: U.S. Department of Health and Human Services, Centers for Disease Control and Prevention, National Center for Environmen tal Health, Division of Laboratory Sciences, 2005b. NCEH Publication No. 05-0570.

Emmons KM, Hammond SK, Fava JL, Velicer WF, Evans JL, Monroe AD. A randomized trial to reduce passive smoke exposure in low-income households with young children. *Pediatrics* 2001;108(1):18–24.

Etzel RA, Balk SJ, editors. *Handbook of Pediatric Environmental Health.* Elk Grove Village (IL): American Academy of Pediatrics, 1999.

Farkas AJ, Gilpin EA, Distefan JM, Pierce JP. The effects of household and workplace smoking restrictions on quitting behaviors. *Tobacco Control.* 1999;8(3):261–5.

Farkas AJ, Gilpin EA, White MM, Pierce JP. Associa tion between household and workplace smoking restrictions and adolescent smoking. *Journal of the American Medical Association.* 2000;284(6):717–22.

Federal Register. U.S. Department of Health and Human Services. Implementation of Pro-Children Act of 1994; notice to prohibit smoking in certain facilities, 59 Fed. Reg. 67713 (1994).

Ferrence R, Timmerman T, Ashley MJ, Northrup D, Brewster J, Cohen J, Leis A, Lovato C, Poland B, Pope M, et al. *Second Hand Smoke in Ontario Homes: Findings from a National Study. Special Reports Series.* Toronto: Ontario Tobacco Research Unit, 2005.

Gehrman CA, Hovell MF. Protecting children from environmental tobacco smoke (ETS) exposure: a critical review. *Nicotine and Tobacco Research.* 2003;5(3):289–301.

Gerlach KK, Shopland DR, Hartman AM, Gibson JT, Pechacek TF. Workplace smoking policies in the United States: results from a national survey of more than 100,000 workers. *Tobacco Control.* 1997;6(3):199–206.

Gilpin EA, Emery SL, Farkas AJ, Distefan JM, White MM, Pierce JP. *The California Tobacco Control Pro¬gram: A Decade of Progress, Results from the California Tobacco Surveys, 1990–1999.* La Jolla (CA): University of California at San Diego, 2001.

Gilpin EA, White MM, Farkas AJ, Pierce JP. Home smoking restrictions: which smokers have them and how they are associated with smoking behavior. *Nicotine and Tobacco Research.* 1999;1(2):153–62.

Hovell MF, Meltzer SB, Wahlgren DR, Matt GE, Hof stetter CR, Jones JA, Meltzer EO, Bernert JT, Pirkle JL. Asthma managementand environmentaltobacco smoke exposure reduction in Latino children: a con trolled trial. *Pediatrics.* 2002;110(5):946–56.

Hovell MF, Zakarian JM, Matt GE, Hofstetter CR, Ber nert JT, Pirkle J. Effects of counselling mothers on their children's exposure to environmental tobacco smoke: randomised controlled trial. *British Medical Journal.* 2000a;321(7257):337–42.

Hovell MF, Zakarian JM, Wahlgren DR, Matt GE. Reducing children's exposure to environmen tal tobacco smoke: the empirical evidence and directions for future research. *Tobacco Control.* 2000b;9(Suppl II):ii40–ii47.

Journal of School Health. School Health Policies and Programs Study (SHPPS) 2000: a summary report. *Journal of School Health.* 2001;71(7):251–350.

Kane MP, Jaen CR, Tumiel LM, Bearman GM, O'Shea RM. Unlimited opportunities for environmental interventions with inner-city asthmatics. *Journal of Asthma.* 1999;36(4):371–9.

Levy DT, Romano E, Mumford EA. Recent trends in home and work smoking bans. *Tobacco Control.* 2004;13(3):258–63.

Mannino DM, Siegel M, Husten C, Rose D, Etzel R. Environmental tobacco smoke exposure and health effects in children: results from the 1991 National Health Interview Survey. *Tobacco Control.* 1996;5(1):13–8.

Mannino DM, Siegel M, Rose, D, Nkuchia J, Etzel R. Environmental tobacco smoke exposure in the home and worksite and health effects in adults:

results from the 1991 National Health Interview Survey. *Tobacco Control.* 1997;6(4):296–305.

Matt GE, Quintana PJE, Hovell MF, Bernert JT, Song S, Novianti N, Juarez T, Floro J, Gehrman C, Gar cia M, et al. Households contaminated by environ mental tobacco smoke: sources of infant exposures. *Tobacco Control.* 2004;13(1):29–37.

McMillen RC, Winickoff JP, Klein JD, Weitzman M. US adult attitudes and practices regarding smoking restrictions and child exposure to environmental tobacco smoke: changes in the social climate from 2000–2001. *Pediatrics.* 2003;112(1):e55–e60.

National Center for Health Statistics. *Plan and operation of the Hispanic Health and Nutrition Examination Survey, 1982–84. Vital and Health Statistics.* Series 1, No. 19. Hyattsville (MD): U.S. Department of Health and Human Services, Public Health Service, National Center for Health Statistics, 1985. DHHS Publication No. (PHS) 85-1321.

National Center for Health Statistics. Health Mea sures in the New 1997 Redesigned National Health Interview Survey (NHIS), April 8, 2004 (updated); <http: / /www.cdc.gov/nchs/about/major/nhis/ hisdesgn.htm>; accessed: June 1, 2004.

National Institute for Occupational Safety and Health. *Environmental Tobacco Smoke in the Workplace: Lung Cancer and Other Health Effects.* Current Intelligence Bulletin 54. Cincinnati: U.S. Department of Health and Human Services, Public Health Service, Cen ters for Disease Control, National Institute for Occupational Safety and Health, Division of Stan dards Development and Technology Transfer, Division of Surveillance, Hazard Evaluations, and Field Studies, 1991. DHHS (NIOSH) Publication No. 91-108.

Nelson DE, Sacks JJ, Addiss DG. Smoking policies of licensed child day-care centers in the United States. *Pediatrics.* 1993;91(2):460–3.

Okah FA, Choi WS, Okuyemi KS, Ahluwalia JS. Effect of children on home smoking restriction by inner- city smokers. *Pediatrics.* 2002;109(2):244–9.

Overpeck MD, Moss AJ. Children's exposure to envi ronmental cigarette smoke before and after birth: health of our nation's children, United States, 1988. *Advance Data.* 1991;202:1–11.

Pirkle JL, Flegal KM, Bernert JT, Brody DJ, Etzel RA, Maurer KR. Exposure of the US population to environmental tobacco smoke: the Third National Health and Nutrition Examination Survey, 1988 to 1991. *Journal of the American Medical Association.* 1996;275(16):1233–40.

Pizacani BA, Martin DP, Stark MJ, Koepsell TD, Thompson B, Diehr P. Household smoking bans: which households have them and do they work? *Preventive Medicine.* 2003;36(1):99–107.

Pizacani BA, Martin DP, Stark MJ, Koepsell TD, Thompson B, Diehr P. A prospective study of household smoking bans and subsequent cessa tion related behaviour: the role of stage of change. *Tobacco Control.* 2004;13(1):23–8.

Pletsch PK. Environmental tobacco smoke exposure among Hispanic women of reproductive age. *Public Health Nursing.* 1994;11(4):229–35.

Pyle SA, Haddock CK, Hymowitz N, Schwab J, Mesh- berg S. Family rules about exposure to environ mental tobacco smoke. *Families, Systems and Health.* 2005;23(1):3–16.

Repace JL, Jinot J, Bayard S, Emmons K, Hammond SK. Air nicotine and saliva cotinine as indicators of workplace passive smoking exposure and risk. *Risk Analysis* 1998;18(1):71–83.

Shopland DR, Gerlach KK, Burns DM, Hartman AM, Gibson JT. State-specific trends in smoke-free workplace policy coverage: the Current Popula tion Survey Tobacco Use Supplement, 1993 to 1999. *Journal of Occupational and Environmental Medicine.* 2001;43(8):680–6.

Smith K. Who's Minding the Kids? Child Care Arrangements. Current Population Reports, P70 70. Washington: U.S. Department of Commerce, Economics and Statistics Administration, U.S. Cen sus Bureau, Fall 1995.

Soliman S, Pollack HA, Warner KE. Decrease in the prevalence of environmental tobacco smoke expo sure in the home during the 1990s in families with children. *American Journal of Public Health.* 2004;94(2):314–20.

Steenland K, Sieber K, Etzel RA, Pechacek T, Maurer K. Exposure to environmental tobacco smoke and risk factors for heart disease among never smokers in the Third National Health and Nutrition Exami nation Survey. *American Journal of Epidemiology.* 1998;147(10):932–9.

Task Force on Community Preventive Services. *The Guide to Community Preventive Services: What Works to Promote Health?* New York: Oxford University Press, 2005.

U.S. Department of Commerce. *The Current Population Survey: Design and Methodology.* Technical Paper No. 40. Washington: U.S. Department of Com merce, U.S. Census Bureau, July 1985.

U.S. Department of Commerce. *Statistical Abstract of the United Status: 2004–2005.* 124th ed. Washington: U.S. Department of Commerce, Economics and Sta tistics Administration, U.S. Census Bureau, 2004.

U.S. Department of Health and Human Services. *The Health Consequences of Involuntary Smoking: A Report of the Surgeon General.* Rockville (MD): U.S. Depart ment of Health and Human Services, Public Health Service, Centers for Disease Control, Center for Health Promotion and Education, Office on Smok ing and Health, 1986. DHHS Publication No. (CDC) 87-8398.

U.S. Department of Health and Human Services. *Reducing the Health Consequences of Smoking: 25 Years of Progress. A Report of the Surgeon General.* Rockville (MD): U.S. Department of Health and Human Services, Public Health Service, Centers for Disease Control, National Center for Chronic Disease Prevention and Health Promotion, Office on Smoking and Health, 1989. DHHS Publication No. (CDC) 89-8411.

U.S. Department of Health and Human Services. *Healthy People 2010: Understanding and Improving Health.* Washington: U.S. Government Printing Office, 2000.

U.S. Department of Health and Human Services. Prog ress Review: Tobacco Use, May 14, 2003; <http: / / www.healthypeople.gov/Data/2010prog/focus27/default.htm>; accessed: May 15, 2006.

U.S. Environmental Protection Agency. *Respiratory Health Effects of Passive Smoking: Lung Cancer and Other Disorders.* Washington: Environmental Pro tection Agency, Office of Research and Develop ment, Office of Air and Radiation, 1992. Publication No. EPA/600/006F.

U.S. Environmental Protection Agency. National Sur vey on Environmental Management of Asthma and Children's Exposure to Environmental Tobacco Smoke [fact sheet]; <http: / /www.epa.gov/smoke free/pdfs/survey_fact_sheet.pdf>; accessed: Octo ber 13, 2005.

A VISION FOR THE FUTURE

This country has experienced a substantial reduction of involuntary exposure to secondhand tobacco smoke in recent decades. Significant reduc tions in the rate of smoking among adults began even earlier. Consequently, about 80 percent of adults are now nonsmokers, and many adults and children can live their daily lives without being exposed to second hand smoke. Nevertheless, involuntary exposure to secondhand smoke remains a serious public health hazard.

The 2006 Surgeon General's report, *The Health Consequences of Involuntary Exposure to Tobacco Smoke* (U.S. Department of Health and Human Services

[USDHHS] 2006) documents the mounting and now substantial evidence characterizing the health risks caused by exposure to secondhand smoke. Multiple major reviews of the evidence have concluded that secondhand smoke is a known human carcinogen, and that exposure to secondhand smoke causes adverse effects, particularly on the cardiovascular system and the respiratory tract and on the health of those exposed, children as well as adults. Unfortunately, reductions in exposure have been slower among young children than among adults during the last decade, as expand ing workplace restrictions now protect the majority of adults while homes remain the most important source of exposure for children.

Clearly, the social norms regarding secondhand smoke have changed dramatically, leading to wide spread support over the past 30 years for a society free of involuntary exposures to tobacco smoke. In the first half of the twentieth century smoking was permitted in almost all public places, including elevators and all types of public transportation. At the time of the 1964 Surgeon General's report on smoking and health (U.S. Department of Health, Education, and Welfare [USDHEW] 1964), many physicians were still smok ers, and the tables in U.S. Public Health Service (PHS) meeting rooms had PHS ashtrays on them. A thick, smoky haze was an accepted part of presentations at large meetings, even at medical conferences and in the hospital environment.

As the adverse health consequences of active smoking became more widely documented in the 1960s, many people began to question whether expo sure of nonsmokers to secondhand smoke also posed a serious health risk. This topic was first addressed in this series of reports by Surgeon General Jesse Steinfeld in the 1972 report to Congress (USDHEW 1972). During the 1970s, policy changes to provide smoke-free environments received more widespread consideration. As the public policy debate grew and expanded in the 1980s, the scientific evidence on the risk of adverse effects from exposure to secondhand smoke was presented in a comprehensive context for the first time by Surgeon General C. Everett Koop in the 1986 report, *The Health Consequences of Involuntary Smoking* (USDHHS 1986).

The ever-increasing momentum for smoke-free indoor environments has been driven by scientific evidence on the health risks of involuntary exposure to secondhand smoke. The 2006 Surgeon General's report (USDHHS 2006) is based on a far larger body of evidence than was available in 1986. The evidence reviewed in the 665 pages of the full report confirms the findings of the 1986 report and adds new causal conclusions. The growing body of data increases sup port for the conclusion that exposure to secondhand smoke causes lung cancer in lifetime nonsmokers. In addition to epidemiologic data, the report presents converging evidence that the mechanisms by which secondhand smoke causes lung cancer are similar to those that cause lung cancer in active smokers. In the context of the risks from active smoking, the lung cancer risk that secondhand smoke exposure poses to nonsmokers is consistent with an extension to involuntary smokers of the dose-response relationship for active smokers.

Cardiovascular effects of even short exposures to secondhand smoke are readily measurable, and the risks for cardiovascular disease from involuntary smoking appear to be about 50 percent less than the risks for active smokers. Although the risks from secondhand smoke exposures are larger than anticipated, research on the mechanisms by which tobacco smoke exposure affects the cardiovascular system supports the plausibility of the findings of epidemiologic studies (the 1986 report did not address cardiovascular disease). The 2006 report also reviews the evidence on the multiple mechanisms by which secondhand smoke injures the respiratory tract and causes sudden infant death syndrome (USDHHS 2006).

Since 1986, the attitude of the public toward and the social norms around secondhand smoke exposure have changed dramatically to reflect a growing viewpoint that the involuntary exposure of nonsmokers to secondhand smoke is unacceptable. As a result, increasingly strict public policies to control involuntary exposure to secondhand smoke have been put in place. The need for restrictions on smoking in enclosed public places is now widely accepted in the United States. A growing number of communities, counties, and states are requiring smoke-free environments for nearly all enclosed public places, including all private worksites, restaurants, bars, and casinos.

As knowledge about the health risks of secondhand smoke exposure grows, investigators continue to identify additional scientific questions.

- Because active smoking is firmly established as a causal factor of cancer for a large number of sites, and because many scientists assert that there may be no threshold for carcinogenesis from tobacco smoke exposure, researchers hypothesize that people who are exposed to secondhand smoke are likely to be at some risk for the same types of cancers that have been established as smoking-related among active smokers.
- The potential risks for stroke and subclinical vascular disease from secondhand smoke exposure require additional research.
- There is a need for additional research on the etiologic relationship between secondhand smoke exposure and several respiratory health outcomes in adults, including respiratory symptoms, declines in lung function, and adult-onset asthma.

- There is also a need for research to further eval uate the adverse reproductive outcomes and childhood respiratory effects from both prenatal and postnatal exposure to secondhand smoke.
- Further research and improved methodologies are also needed to advance an understanding of the potential effects on cognitive, behavioral, and physical development that might be related to early exposures to secondhand smoke.

As these and other research questions are addressed, the scientific literature documenting the adverse health effects of exposure to secondhand smoke will expand. Over the past 40 years since the release of the landmark 1964 report of the Surgeon

General's Advisory Committee on Smoking and Health (USDHEW 1964), researchers have compiled an ever-growing list of adverse health effects caused by exposure to tobacco smoke, with evidence that active smoking causes damage to virtually every organ of the body (USDHHS 2004). Similarly, since the 1986 report (USDHHS 1986), the number of adverse health effects caused by exposure to secondhand smoke has also expanded. Following the format of the electronic database released with the 2004 report, the research findings supporting the conclusions in the 2006 report are accessible in a database that can be found at http://www.cdc.gov/tobacco. With an expanding base of scientific knowledge, the list of adverse health effects caused by exposure to secondhand smoke will likely increase.

Biomarker data from the 2005 *Third National Report on Human Exposure to Environmental Chemicals* document great progress since the 1986 report in reducing the involuntary exposure of nonsmokers to secondhand smoke (CDC 2005). Between the late 1980s and 2002, the median cotinine level (a metabolite of nicotine) among nonsmokers declined by more than 70 percent. Nevertheless, many challenges remain to maintain the momentum toward universal smoke-free environments.

- First, there is a need to continue and even improve the surveillance of sources and levels of exposure to secondhand smoke. The data from the 2005 exposure report show that median cotinine levels among children are more than twice those of nonsmoking adults, and non- Hispanic Blacks have levels more than twice those of Mexican Americans and non-Hispanic Whites (CDC 2005). The multiple factors related to these disparities in median cotinine levels among nonsmokers need to be identified and addressed.

- Second, the data from the 2005 exposure report suggest that the scientific community should sustain the current momentum to reduce exposures of nonsmokers to secondhand smoke (CDC 2005). Research reviewed in this report indicates that policies creating completely smoke- free environments are the most economical and efficient approaches to providing this protection. Additionally, neither central heating, ventilating, and air conditioning systems nor separately ventilated rooms control exposures to secondhand smoke.
- Unfortunately, data from the 2005 exposure report also emphasized that young children remain an exposed population (CDC 2005). However, more evidence is needed on the most effective strategies to promote voluntary changes in smoking norms and practices in homes and private automobiles.
- Finally, data on the health consequences of secondhand smoke exposures emphasize the importance of the role of health care professionals in this issue. They must assume a greater, more active involvement in reducing exposures, particularly for susceptible groups.

The findings and recommendations of this report can be extended to other countries and are supportive of international efforts to address the health effects of smoking and secondhand smoke exposure. There is an international consensus that exposure to secondhand smoke poses significant public health risks. The Frame work Convention on Tobacco Control recognizes that protecting nonsmokers from involuntary exposures to secondhand smoke in public places should be an integral part of comprehensive national tobacco con trol policies and programs. Recent changes in national policies in countries such as Italy and Ireland reflect this growing international awareness of the need for additional protection of nonsmokers from involuntary exposures to secondhand smoke.

When this series of reports began in 1964, the majority of men and a substantial proportion of women were smokers, and most nonsmokers inevitably must have been involuntary smokers. With the release of the 1986 report, Surgeon General Koop noted that "the right of smokers to smoke ends where their behavior affects the health and well-being of others" (USDHHS 1986, p. xii). As understanding increases regarding health consequences from even brief expo sures to secondhand smoke, it becomes even clearer that the health of nonsmokers overall, and particu larly the health of children, individuals with exist ing heart and lung problems, and other vulnerable populations, requires a higher priority and greater protection.

Together, the 2004 and 2006 reports of the Surgeon General (USDHHS 2004, 2006), document the extraordinary threat to the nation's health from active and involuntary smoking. The recent reduc tions in exposures of nonsmokers to secondhand smoke represent significant progress, but involun tary exposures persist in many settings and environ ments. More evidence is needed to understand why this progress has not been equally shared across all populations and in all parts of this nation. Some states (California, Connecticut, Delaware, Maine, Massachusetts, New York, Rhode Island, and Wash ington) have met the *Healthy People 2010* objectives (USDHHS 2000) that protect against involuntary exposures to secondhand smoke through recom mended policies, regulations, and laws, while many other parts of this nation have not (USDHHS 2000). Evidence presented in this report suggests that these disparities in levels of protection can be reduced or eliminated. Sustained progress toward a society free of involuntary exposures to secondhand smoke should remain a national public health priority.

REFERENCES

Centers for Disease Control and Prevention. *Third National Report on Human Exposure to Environmental Chemicals.* Atlanta: U.S. Department of Health and Human Services, Centers for Disease Control and Prevention, National Center for Environmental Health, 2005. NCEH Publication No. 05-0570.

U.S. Department of Health and Human Services. *The Health Consequences of Involuntary Smoking. A Report of the Surgeon General.* Rockville (MD): U.S. Department of Health and Human Services, Public Health Service, Centers for Disease Control, Cen ter for Health Promotion and Education, Office on Smoking and Health, 1986. DHHS Publication No. (CDC) 87-8398.

U.S. Department of Health and Human Services. *Healthy People 2010: Understanding and Improving Health.* Washington: U.S. Government Printing Office, 2000.

U.S. Department of Health and Human Services. *The Health Consequences of Smoking: A Report of the Surgeon General.* Atlanta: U.S. Department of Health and Human Services, Centers for Disease Control and Prevention, National Center for Chronic Dis ease Prevention and Health Promotion, Office on Smoking and Health, 2004.

U.S. Department of Health and Human Services. *The Health Consequences of Involuntary Exposure to Tobacco Smoke: A Report of the Surgeon General.* Atlanta: U.S. Department of Health and Human Services, Centers for Disease Control and Prevention, National Center for Chronic Disease Prevention and Health Promotion, Office on Smoking and Health, 2006.

U.S. Department of Health, Education, and Welfare. *Smoking and Health: Report of the Advisory Committee to the Surgeon General of the Public Health Service.* Washington: U.S. Department of Health, Education, and Welfare, Public Health Service, Center for Disease Control, 1964. PHS Publication No. 1103.

U.S. Department of Health, Education, and Welfare. *The Health Consequences of Smoking: A Report of the Surgeon General: 1972.* Washington: U.S. Department of Health, Education, and Welfare, Public Health Service, Health Services and Mental Health Administration, 1972. DHEW Publication No. (HSM) 72-7516.

INDEX

A

abnormalities, 52, 65, 100, 102, 114, 115
abortion, 48, 52, 53, 71, 77, 87
absorption, 7
abstinence, 131
acetylcholine, 126
acid, 96
activation, 48, 68, 96
active smokers, 50, 144, 152
acute, 11, 33, 40, 75, 89, 100, 103, 104, 105, 108, 110, 116, 121, 126, 127
addiction, 146
adducts, 37, 50, 68, 76, 77, 87
adenocarcinoma, 68
adenoidectomy, 105, 116
adjustment, 56, 57, 70, 99, 100
administration, 68, 92
adolescence, 97, 115
adolescents, 36, 132, 134, 140
adrenal gland, 69
adrenal glands, 69
adult, 18, 26, 40, 89, 130, 131, 132, 133, 134, 148, 152
adulthood, 115, 125
adults, vii, viii, 1, 2, 3, 4, 6, 7, 8, 9, 11, 18, 19, 23, 25, 26, 27, 28, 34, 35, 36, 37, 39, 40, 42, 48, 57, 58, 64, 113, 121, 130, 131, 134, 135, 143, 144, 147, 150, 151, 152, 153
age, vii, 17, 18, 19, 20, 27, 29, 30, 32, 51, 52, 53, 55, 56, 60, 65, 70, 77, 79, 90, 91, 97, 98, 99, 100, 103, 106, 107, 108, 110, 113, 114, 116, 117, 120, 121, 122, 126, 133, 134, 135, 136, 137, 141, 149
agents, 82
aggregation, 110
aging, 115
air, 5, 10, 11, 17, 36, 38, 41, 96, 97, 110, 125, 126, 135, 143, 144, 154
air pollution, 96, 110, 126
air quality, 41
airflow obstruction, 96, 118
airway inflammation, 96, 97
airways, 56, 91, 93, 110, 114, 115, 124
alcohol, 51, 52, 53, 64
alcohol consumption, 51, 52
alkylating agents, 82
allergen challenge, 96, 127
allergens, 96, 112
allergic asthma, 109
allergic rhinitis, 112
allergy, 113, 117, 123, 126
alpha, 78
alters, 34, 65, 83, 125
alveoli, 92, 114
ambient air, 96
amniotic, 68, 75, 93, 121
amniotic fluid, 68, 75, 93, 121

analysis of variance, 136
animal models, 55, 56, 93
animal studies, 48, 49, 52, 65, 67, 68
animals, 62, 69
antigen (s), 94, 95
apoptotic, 80
appendix, 90
application, 15, 40
arachidonic acid, 96
Arbacia punctulata, 80
argument, 61
aromatic hydrocarbons, 52
artery, 75
aspiration, 80
assessment, 6, 8, 15, 39, 48, 57, 66, 74, 99, 106, 113
asthma, vii, 1, 3, 8, 9, 11, 16, 25, 29, 33, 39, 84, 90, 94, 95, 100, 102, 106, 107, 108, 109, 110, 111, 117, 118, 120, 122, 123, 124, 125, 126, 131, 133, 135, 137, 142, 152
asthmatic children, 138
asthmatic symptoms, 110
astrocytoma, 79
atmosphere, 5
atopic dermatitis, 124
atopy, 95, 96, 113, 123, 126, 128
attacks, 110, 118
attitudes, ix, 36, 40, 129, 148
automobiles, 34, 154
autonomic pathways, 65
autopsy, 56
awareness, 138, 154

B

bacteria, 96, 101
bacterial, 96, 127
barrier, 92
barriers, 144
behavior, 7, 138, 154
behavior modification, 138
behavioral problems, 66, 73
bias, 7, 10, 57, 69, 101, 102, 104
binding, 92

biomarker, 16, 36, 40
biomarkers, 6, 16, 50
biomass, 101
birth, 9, 29, 40, 45, 54, 56, 60, 61, 62, 64, 69, 70, 72, 77, 78, 79, 80, 81, 91, 93, 94, 95, 100, 101, 102, 107, 112, 114, 115, 117, 120, 122, 123, 124, 148
birth weight, 9, 45, 54, 56, 60, 61, 62, 64, 72, 77, 79, 81, 91, 93, 120, 123, 124
births, 60
birthweight, 38, 80, 87
blastocyst, 49
blood, 17, 60, 65, 68, 69, 76, 77, 78, 80, 87, 91, 94, 95, 111, 119, 124, 125
blood flow, 60, 65, 91, 125
blood vessels, 78
body mass index, 51
body size, 100
Boolean logic, 16
boys, 96
brain, 48, 56, 65, 69, 70, 71, 73, 75, 77, 78, 80, 82, 83
brain damage, 65
brain development, 77
brain tumor, 69, 70, 71, 73, 78, 82
breast milk, 79
breathing, 6, 38, 55, 127, 145
breathlessness, 106, 107, 116
bronchiolitis, 124
bronchitis, 76, 103, 109, 120, 128
bronchoalveolar lavage, 95, 96
buildings, 11, 23, 36, 142, 144
burn, 10
burns, 131
buses, 6, 16

C

cadmium, 52
caffeine, 53
caliber, 93, 110
cancer, 6, 7, 8, 9, 11, 50, 53, 67, 69, 70, 71, 73, 74, 145, 151, 152
capacity, 93, 99, 128
carbon, 5, 52

Index

carbon monoxide, 5, 52
carcinogen, 8, 37, 38, 76, 82, 151
carcinogenesis, 7, 68, 81, 82, 84, 152
carcinogenic, 69
carcinogenicity, 7, 8
carcinogens, 6, 67, 82, 84
cardiovascular disease, 6, 152
cardiovascular system, 11, 151, 152
caregiver, 103
caregivers, ix
catecholamines, 93, 121
cation, 59, 85
causal interpretation, 107
causal relationship, 51, 53, 54, 55, 58, 60, 62, 63, 66, 67, 70, 71, 72, 73, 103, 105, 107, 111, 113, 115, 116, 117, 118
causality, 9, 54, 74, 111
causation, 115
cell, 48, 56, 61, 68, 74, 83, 86, 94, 96
cell signaling, 83
cellular immunity, 94
central nervous system, 65
cervical cancer, 50
cervix, 83
child development, 45
childbearing, 30
cholinergic, 92
chromosomal abnormalities, 52
chronic obstructive pulmonary disease, 6
chronic respiratory morbidity, 89
cigarette smoke, 5, 10, 36, 40, 49, 62, 68, 82, 84, 87, 93, 96, 110, 113, 119, 121, 122, 123, 125, 126, 148
cigarette smokers, 36, 113, 122
cigarette smoking, 36, 50, 76, 78, 81, 82, 83, 123, 127
cigarettes, 5, 26, 27, 29, 30, 61, 68, 96, 107, 131, 137
civilian, 17
classification, 100, 101
cleaning, 11, 143, 144
cleavage, 49
clinical diagnosis, 118
clinics, 50
cocaine, 83

coffee, 86
cognitive, 48, 64, 65, 66, 67, 72, 74, 153
cognitive development, 48, 64, 65, 74
cognitive function, 66, 67, 72
cognitive process, 48, 65
cohort, 78, 90, 97, 98, 101, 108, 109, 110, 113, 114, 115, 126, 140, 141
collagen, 92, 93, 125
colony-stimulating factor, 95
combined effect, 47
combustion, 9, 101
common symptoms, 106
communities, 102, 142, 152
community, 29, 34, 121, 136, 154
compilation, 6
compliance, 141, 143
complications, 59, 75
components, 5, 6, 10, 29, 30, 52, 65, 68, 91, 92, 96, 105, 112, 144
composition, 10, 16, 128
compounds, 82
concentration, 16, 19, 26, 27, 31, 32, 33, 47, 61, 78, 82, 135
conception, 49, 50, 51, 75, 78
concrete, 138
conditioning, 154
conductor, 77
confidence, 97, 101
confidence interval, 97
conflict, 50
confounders, 51, 56, 57
confounding variables, 99, 103
consensus, 100, 154
constraints, 111
consumption, 38, 51, 52, 53, 131
contaminants, 144
contamination, 26, 122, 135
control, 7, 11, 36, 57, 64, 70, 78, 79, 82, 90, 92, 98, 102, 108, 109, 126, 129, 134, 135, 137, 139, 144, 152, 154
control group, 137
controlled trials, 139
coronary heart disease, 11
correlation, 31, 64, 69
correlation coefficient, 31

cortisol, 47, 93
cotinine, 2, 3, 6, 16, 17, 18, 19, 20, 22, 24, 26, 27, 28, 30, 32, 34, 36, 37, 38, 40, 51, 52, 57, 59, 61, 69, 78, 79, 81, 82, 100, 101, 107, 135, 137, 145, 149, 153
cough, 90, 97, 106, 107, 116
counseling, 136, 137, 138, 139
couples, 76
covalent, 77
coverage, 9, 42, 130, 149
critical period, 83, 94
cross-sectional, 98, 99, 100, 106, 107, 109, 113, 114, 115, 141
customers, 43
cyanide, 52
cytokine, 94, 95
cytokines, 95, 96, 124

D

daily living, 82
data collection, 29
data set, 80
database, 46, 153
death, vii, 1, 3, 8, 11, 47, 54, 55, 58, 72, 74, 75, 79, 80, 82, 93, 121, 123, 152
death rate, 55
deaths, 8, 54, 74, 80, 103, 145
decisions, 4
defects, 48, 63, 78
deficits, 65, 67
definition, 10, 25, 132
delivery, 54, 59, 60, 61, 72, 114
demographic factors, 53
demographics, 134, 140
density, 50, 86, 93
dermatitis, 124
detection, 18, 22, 24, 119
developed countries, 100, 103
developing brain, 48
developing countries, 101, 126
developmental process, 47, 48
deviation, 93
differentiation, 48, 64
diffusion, 128, 136

discomfort, 5
diseases, 8, 89, 97, 104, 106, 112
distribution, 18
dose-response relationship, 7, 52, 74, 99, 152
dosimetry, 7
draft, 15
drug use, 70
duration, 23, 33, 137
dust, 96, 124, 125, 135

E

ears, 109
eating, 33
eczema, 112
educational programs, 28
effusion, 104, 105, 116
egg, 52
elastin, 93
embryo, 48, 49, 52, 77, 78
employers, 132
endocrine, 92
endotoxins, 96
enrollment, 140
entertainment, 143
environment, 6, 10, 63, 64, 78, 86, 92, 94, 96, 97, 142, 151
environmental factors, 75, 111, 115
environmental tobacco, 9, 10, 15, 16, 36, 37, 38, 39, 40, 41, 42, 43, 76, 77, 78, 79, 82, 83, 87, 90, 123, 147, 148, 149
enzymes, 86
eosinophil count, 96
eosinophilia, 96, 125
eosinophils, 95
epidemiologic studies, 50, 51, 69, 89, 101, 106
epidemiology, 43, 121
epithelium, 126
erythropoietin, 61, 78, 79, 80
estradiol, 49
ethnic groups, 139
ethnicity, 18, 20, 21, 27, 143
etiologic factor, 102

etiology, 52, 62, 71, 100, 105, 111
evening, 33
excitability, 97
expert, iv
eyes, 40

F

failure, 49, 103
familial, 79, 110
familial aggregation, 110
family, 39, 84, 98, 103, 121, 124, 126, 137, 141
family factors, 121
family history, 84, 124, 126
federal government, 136
feedback, 136
females, 30, 145
fertility, 45, 47, 49, 50, 51, 71, 76, 80
fertilization, 49, 50, 77, 78, 80, 82, 84, 87
fetal, 45, 47, 48, 52, 60, 61, 62, 68, 75, 77, 78, 79, 80, 82, 84, 91, 92, 120, 123, 124, 125, 127
fetal growth, 45, 60, 91, 92
fetal growth retardation, 61
fetus, 10, 30, 47, 48, 52, 55, 60, 65, 84, 91, 92, 93, 114, 115, 118
fetuses, 29, 37, 76, 93, 95
fever, 52
fiber (s), 97, 124
fires, 131
flex, 98
flow, 60, 65, 75, 91, 93, 99, 114, 120, 125, 126
flow rate, 99, 114
fluid, 49, 50, 68, 86, 93, 95, 96, 121
focusing, 2, 45
follicular, 49, 50, 86
follicular fluid, 49, 50, 86
food, 33
fuel, 101
funding, 141

G

gamete, 50
gamete intrafallopian transfer, 50
gametogenesis, 80
gases, 9, 128
gender, 18, 20, 99, 100, 133, 143, 145
gene, 48, 63, 69, 78, 83, 86, 94, 97, 114, 125
gene expression, 48, 125
generation, 86
genes, 63, 92
genetics, 110
genomic, 69
gestation, 48, 52, 59, 60, 75, 78, 93, 114
gestational age, 53, 60
glioma, 75
globulin, 95
government, 28, 129, 132, 136
gram-negative bacteria, 96
grandparents, 133
graph, 7
greed, 130
groups, 23, 25, 29, 46, 64, 100, 132, 135, 137, 139, 143, 145, 154
growth, vii, 1, 3, 8, 11, 45, 47, 48, 60, 67, 73, 78, 83, 89, 90, 91, 92, 97, 113, 114, 115
growth factor, 78, 83
growth hormone, 47
guanine, 69
guidelines, 139, 142, 144

H

harm, 5
harmful effects, 3, 7
haze, 151
health care, 136, 137, 139, 141, 154
health care professionals, 154
health care sector, 139
health effects, 3, 6, 8, 9, 15, 26, 30, 40, 89, 90, 91, 97, 99, 117, 129, 144, 147, 153, 154

health problems, viii
heart, 5, 6, 8, 9, 11, 83, 131, 145, 149, 154
heart disease, 8, 9, 11, 131, 145, 149
heating, 154
height, 67, 73
hemoglobin, 38, 76
heterogeneity, 101, 104, 106
high risk, 82
high school, 142
high temperature, 9
hormone, 47
hormones, 47
hospital, 89, 122, 151
hospitality, 143
hospitalization, 120
hospitals, 143
house dust, 124
household, 2, 4, 19, 26, 27, 28, 29, 42, 47, 49, 57, 58, 79, 96, 98, 99, 100, 103, 107, 109, 131, 132, 134, 135, 136, 138, 139, 140, 146, 149
households, 25, 26, 28, 36, 37, 57, 102, 109, 129, 132, 133, 135, 136, 140, 146, 149
housing, 101
human, 8, 39, 48, 49, 52, 55, 65, 68, 76, 77, 78, 80, 81, 92, 93, 95, 119, 151
human exposure, 39
humans, 49, 62, 95
hydro, 52
hygienic, 131
hypoplasia, 92, 120
hypothesis, 61, 92, 109, 111
hypoxia, 48, 56, 60, 61, 65, 80, 91, 123

I

immune function, 94, 97
immune system, 91, 94
immunity, 94, 121
immunization, 137
immunoglobulin, 94, 113, 117
immunophenotype, 94, 106, 112
immunophenotypes, 112

in utero, 29, 37, 76, 77, 92, 93, 94, 95, 97, 100, 106, 114, 115, 118
in vitro, 50, 82, 83, 86, 87
in vitro fertilization, 50, 82, 87
in vivo, 83
incidence, 7, 8, 99, 100, 102, 106, 107, 108, 109, 110, 111, 118
inclusion, 5, 16, 102
income, 2, 28, 31, 37, 132, 133, 134, 135, 136, 146
incomes, 35, 133
indication, 78, 100, 109
indicators, 6, 40, 80, 118, 149
indices, 98, 99, 120, 123
induction, 49, 94, 110
industry, 32, 143
infancy, 70, 73, 89, 90, 91, 97, 99, 100, 109, 110, 112, 113, 118, 119, 126
infant mortality, 45, 54, 58, 74
infant mortality rate, 54, 74
infants, 1, 3, 7, 27, 38, 40, 45, 48, 54, 56, 57, 58, 61, 68, 69, 74, 78, 82, 84, 87, 89, 91, 92, 93, 95, 97, 101, 102, 103, 104, 110, 111, 112, 116, 117, 121, 122, 123, 126, 135
infection, 97, 100, 102, 109, 110, 121, 122, 123
infections, vii, 1, 3, 8, 9, 11, 56, 100, 102, 103, 110, 118, 121, 123, 124, 126, 128
infertility, 47, 49, 50, 51, 75, 76, 79, 84
inflammation, 96, 97, 115
inflammatory, 94, 96, 127
inflammatory response, 94, 127
inflammatory responses, 94
inhalation, 9, 10, 96
initiation, 110, 142
initiation rates, 142
injury, iv, 47, 102
institutions, 16
insults, 48
interaction, 78, 86, 136
interactions, 63, 94, 97
interferon, 94, 95, 119, 121
interferon gamma, 94, 95
interleukin, 95, 119

interpretation, 30, 90, 107
interstitial, 93, 128
interval, 6, 17, 22, 24, 50, 97
intervention, 130, 135, 136, 137
interviews, 17, 29, 51, 53, 58, 69, 133
intrauterine growth retardation, 60
intravenously, 68
Investigations, 49
involuntary smoke, 154
ionization, 145
irritation, 6, 56, 97
isolation, 144

J

junior high, 142
junior high school, 142

K

kindergarten, 141
kinetics, 76

L

labor, 59
laboratory method, 18
land, 31
language, 10, 98
large-scale, 139
laws, 36, 141, 155
lead, 5, 34, 47, 48, 52, 59, 60, 61, 65, 68, 91, 92, 93, 115, 135, 143, 144
learning, 65, 138
lectin, 93
legislation, 129, 141
lesions, 81
leukemia, 69, 70, 73
life style, 34
lifespan, 80
lifestyles, 142
lifetime, 7, 18, 53, 144, 151
likelihood, 100

limitation, 60, 141
limitations, 91
links, 117
lipid, 83
lipid peroxidation, 83
lipopolysaccharide, 127
location, 16, 23, 143
long period, 139
long-term, 36, 65, 89, 97, 109, 118
losses, 52, 53
low birthweight, 80
low risk, 110
lower respiratory tract infection, 8, 123
low-income, 28, 31, 37, 135, 136, 146
lung, vii, 1, 3, 5, 6, 7, 8, 9, 11, 69, 89, 90, 91, 92, 93, 94, 96, 97, 100, 102, 103, 106, 112, 113, 114, 115, 117, 119, 120, 122, 123, 124, 125, 127, 145, 151, 152, 154
lung cancer, 6, 7, 8, 11, 145, 151
lung disease, 5, 6, 89, 116
lung function, 90, 92, 100, 102, 113, 114, 115, 117, 122, 123, 125, 127, 152
lungs, 10, 97
luteinizing hormone, 47
lymphocytes, 77
lymphoma, 69, 70
lymphomas, 69, 70, 73

M

macrophage, 94, 119, 121
magnetic, iv
mainstream, 5, 7, 9, 65, 84, 87, 93, 94, 96
mainstream smoke, 5, 6, 7, 9, 65, 84, 93, 96
major histocompatibility complex, 94
males, 145
mass spectrometry, 145
maternal age, 52, 53, 56
maturation, 92, 97, 114, 123
measures, 19, 57, 58, 66, 74, 77, 90, 95, 98, 100, 104, 106, 107, 112, 115, 129, 136, 138
meconium, 101, 124

media, 104, 105, 116, 121, 123, 127, 136, 139
median, 19, 31, 32, 135, 153
mediators, 123
medication, 86
medications, viii
membranes, 78, 86
memory, 48, 65
memory deficits, 65
men, 34, 50, 66, 144, 154
menstrual cycle, 49
messages, 142
meta analysis, 62, 75
meta-analysis, 8, 9, 50, 56, 62, 80, 86, 87, 94, 99, 100, 102, 104, 107, 112, 114
metabolic, 27, 92
metabolism, 17, 76, 82
metabolite, 6, 16, 87, 153
metabolites, 52, 68, 96, 121
metropolitan area, 127
mice, 95, 121, 125
microbial, 100
microenvironments, 23, 34
micrograms, 31
middle ear infection, 9
middle schools, 142
middle-aged, 36
milk, 79
miscarriages, 52, 53
modeling, 39, 57
moisture content, 10
molecules, 96
momentum, 151, 153, 154
monkeys, 83, 92, 125
monocytes, 119
morbidity, 89, 103
morphometric, 120
mortality, 45, 54, 58, 72, 74, 80, 81, 86, 121, 145
mortality rate, 54, 74
mothers, 26, 29, 55, 56, 61, 64, 68, 69, 70, 76, 87, 93, 95, 102, 103, 122, 123, 138, 147
movement, 92
mucus, 50, 59, 61, 81, 82, 83

multiple factors, 28, 153
multiplication, 99
multivariate, 70, 97, 104
murine model, 126
muscle, 93, 121
mutations, 69, 74, 77

N

nation, 2, 18, 19, 26, 40, 148, 149, 155
natural, 50, 51, 78, 105, 109, 116
neonatal, 45, 54, 55, 72, 76, 81, 83, 92, 95, 121, 128
neonates, 60, 112, 119
neoplasia, 83
neoplasms, 69
nerve, 97
nervous system, vii, 3, 65
neural function, 48, 65
neurobehavioral, 56
neurotoxic, 55
neutrophilia, 122
neutrophils, 96
nicotine, 6, 16, 17, 18, 30, 31, 32, 33, 38, 39, 40, 48, 49, 51, 52, 55, 57, 59, 60, 61, 65, 69, 75, 78, 79, 80, 81, 82, 83, 87, 91, 92, 125, 135, 136, 149, 153
nitric oxide, 94
nitrogen, 6
nitrogen oxides, 6
nitrosamines, 59
nonsmokers, ix, 5, 6, 7, 8, 9, 10, 11, 15, 17, 18, 19, 20, 24, 28, 31, 32, 33, 34, 35, 36, 38, 41, 42, 50, 52, 53, 54, 56, 59, 75, 80, 81, 82, 93, 130, 131, 134, 143, 144, 150, 151, 152, 153, 154, 155
non-smokers, 39
non-smokers, 120
norms, 132, 139, 142, 151, 152, 154
nurse, 137
nursing, 16, 25
nursing home, 16, 25

O

obstruction, 96, 118, 125
obstructive lung disease, 89
occupational, 36, 52
odds ratio, 50, 98
oil, 69
older adults, 19, 36
olive, 69
olive oil, 69
oocyte, 47
oogenesis, 80
oral, 63, 78, 80, 81, 86, 87
organ, 97, 153
organizations, 135
otitis media, 104, 105, 116, 121, 123, 127
outcome of interest, 98, 137
outcome relationship, 103
outpatient, 110
oviduct, 49, 83
ovulation, 49, 86
ovum, 52
ownership, 141
oxide, 94
oxides, 6
oxygen, 60, 65, 114

P

pairing, 16
pancreas, 69
paper, 9, 99
parenchyma, 93
parental smoking, 6, 8, 28, 69, 76, 89, 90, 94, 98, 99, 100, 101, 102, 103, 104, 105, 106, 107, 108, 109, 110, 111, 112, 113, 114, 115, 116, 117, 118, 120, 123, 124, 126, 137
parents, 1, 3, 6, 11, 28, 89, 95, 98, 100, 103, 104, 105, 107, 108, 109, 110, 114, 125, 130, 136, 138, 139
particle mass, 39
particles, 9, 10, 41, 42, 97, 119
particulate matter, 6, 30

passive, 5, 6, 7, 9, 16, 31, 37, 38, 40, 46, 75, 76, 77, 78, 79, 81, 87, 102, 119, 120, 121, 122, 126, 136, 146, 149
passive smoke, 37, 75, 81, 87, 146
passive smokers, 75, 81, 87
paternal, 46, 47, 49, 50, 51, 53, 54, 57, 70, 71, 74, 89, 98, 102, 107, 109, 117
pathogens, 102
pathways, 65, 94, 97
patients, 39, 51, 86
pediatric, 79, 139
pediatrician, viii, 137
peer, 143
percentile, 18, 31, 60
performance, 66, 114, 145
perinatal, 46, 81, 86
permeability, 96, 122
permit, 144
peroxidation, 83
persistent asthma, 110
personal, 23, 29, 31, 38, 40, 41, 42
pets, 119
phenotype, 86, 95, 97, 100, 101, 106, 110, 111, 113, 118
phenotypes, 94, 95, 100, 111, 118
phenotypic, 101
phlegm, 76, 90, 106, 107, 116, 120
physicians, viii, 151
pig, 97
pigs, 48, 65, 97, 119, 124, 126
placenta, 59, 61, 65, 77, 78, 81, 95
placenta previa, 59, 81
placental, 68, 80, 81, 92
placental barrier, 92
plasma, 79
plastic, 81
plausibility, 7, 49, 59, 115, 152
play, viii, 50, 69, 76, 102, 139
pneumonia, viii, 101, 103, 127
policymakers, 15
pollutants, 39
pollution, 16, 96, 110, 126
polycyclic aromatic hydrocarbon, 52
polymorphism, 78
polymorphisms, 79, 86

polysaccharide, 122
population, 2, 8, 16, 17, 18, 19, 24, 25, 29, 32, 36, 38, 42, 43, 58, 78, 82, 101, 137, 140, 145, 148, 154
population group, 2, 29
ports, 118
postnatal exposure, 26, 30, 55, 58, 69, 70, 71, 73, 91, 93, 103, 106, 107, 109, 115, 118, 153
postpartum, 48, 56, 57, 58, 64
postpartum period, 48
poverty, 26, 133
power, 53, 69, 74, 111
predictors, 2, 27, 40, 141
preference, 10, 95
pregnant, 29, 30, 31, 40, 43, 51, 62, 68, 69, 78, 82, 91, 92, 93, 104, 107, 131
pregnant women, 29, 30, 31, 40, 51, 78, 82, 91, 104, 131
premature death, 3, 11
premature labor, 59
prematurity, 91
prenatal care, 74
preschool, 76, 106, 117
preschool children, 76
pressure, 144, 145
preterm delivery, 54, 59, 60, 61, 72
preterm infants, 93, 122
prevention, 105
primary care, 136
primates, 82
prisons, 16
private, 131, 152, 154
probability, 17, 49, 59
production, 47, 61, 76, 94, 120
prognosis, 100, 107, 108, 110, 126
program, 80, 134
programming, 92
prolactin, 47
promote, 2, 28, 94, 95, 134, 136, 154
property, iv, 142
prostaglandin, 96
protection, 43, 154, 155
protein, 48, 61
protocol, 32
protocols, 17
provocation, 110
public, 4, 6, 7, 9, 15, 16, 23, 25, 28, 31, 32, 34, 35, 118, 129, 130, 135, 138, 145, 146, 150, 151, 152, 154, 155
public awareness, 138
public health, ix, 6, 7, 9, 15, 32, 35, 118, 135, 150, 154, 155
public policy, 7, 34, 151
pyrene, 50, 87

Q

questionnaire, 40, 51
questionnaires, 15, 16, 26

R

race, 17, 18, 20, 27, 54, 70, 133
random, 57, 99, 101, 102, 133
range, viii, 8, 28, 30, 33, 56, 58, 97, 107, 112
rat, 87, 92, 128
rats, 48, 65, 82, 83, 92, 93
reactivity, 90, 112
recall, 69
receptors, 92, 97, 122, 126
recognition, 122
recurrence, 108
red blood cell, 60, 76, 87, 94
red blood cell count, 60
red blood cells, 76, 87, 94
reduced lung function, 113
reduction, 1, 50, 60, 61, 62, 72, 79, 91, 92, 103, 113, 116, 136, 147, 150
refining, 138
regional, 34, 83
regular, viii, 96, 133, 141
regulation, 48, 94, 130
regulations, 43, 143, 155
reinforcement, 138
relapse, 140
relationship, 7, 45, 51, 53, 54, 55, 58, 60, 62, 63, 66, 67, 70, 71, 72, 73, 77, 99,

100, 103, 105, 107, 108, 111, 113, 115, 116, 117, 118, 123, 125, 140, 152
relationships, 7, 52, 71, 74, 112, 115, 140
relatives, 133
renal, 68
rent, 118
reproduction, 49, 50, 76, 84
reproductive age, 51, 149
research, 6, 8, 10, 15, 16, 46, 53, 58, 60, 66, 67, 71, 74, 92, 97, 100, 102, 110, 118, 120, 130, 137, 138, 139, 147, 152, 153
research design, 130
researchers, 6, 16, 17, 18, 28, 48, 50, 57, 58, 60, 61, 62, 64, 90, 93, 95, 114, 141, 152, 153
resistance, 100
respiration, 92
respiratory, vii, 1, 3, 6, 7, 8, 9, 11, 40, 42, 46, 56, 68, 79, 84, 89, 90, 91, 92, 93, 94, 97, 100, 102, 103, 105, 106, 108, 110, 116, 117, 118, 119, 120, 121, 122, 123, 124, 125, 126, 128, 151, 152, 153
respiratory rate, 92
respiratory syncytial virus, 122
responsiveness, 94, 95, 118, 121, 123, 124, 126, 128
restaurant, 40, 43
restaurants, 16, 23, 25, 32, 33, 34, 35, 38, 39, 143, 152
retardation, 60, 61, 66
retention, 66
returns, 9, 10
rhinitis, 112
risk assessment, 8, 106, 113
risk factors, 39, 55, 57, 58, 70, 79, 100, 122, 125, 127, 149
risks, vii, ix, 1, 7, 8, 38, 58, 70, 71, 74, 77, 135, 144, 151, 152, 154
robustness, 107
rodents, 82
rural, 28, 39

S

safety, 131, 145
saliva, 40, 69, 78, 149
sample, 17, 18, 28, 53, 63, 78
sampling, 31, 32
school, 23, 39, 90, 98, 100, 106, 107, 108, 116, 117, 120, 140, 141, 142, 146
school enrollment, 140
scientific community, 154
scientific knowledge, 153
scientists, 152
sea urchin, 52, 80
search, 16, 17, 46, 98, 102
searches, 47, 90, 98
secondary schools, 141
selectivity, 83
self-efficacy, 138
self-help, 136
self-report, 18, 27, 28, 77, 98, 136, 137, 145
semen, 51, 82
sensitivity, 123
sensitization, 90, 94, 95, 111, 112, 121, 125
series, 9, 90, 113, 151, 154
serum, 17, 18, 19, 20, 22, 24, 26, 27, 28, 30, 32, 36, 38, 61, 75, 79, 86, 95, 112, 122, 123, 125, 145
services, iv, 141, 142
severe asthma, vii, 1, 3, 11, 109
severity, 100, 102, 107, 108, 109, 110, 118
sharing, 56, 58
sheep, 94
short-term, 65
siblings, 124
sidestream smoke, 9, 48, 52, 62, 65, 94, 96, 97
signaling, 83
sinus, 39
sinusitis, 39
sites, 9, 25, 32, 152
skills, 138
skin, 95, 112
sleep, 77

smoking cessation, 104, 136, 137
smooth muscle, 93, 121
social class, 64, 100
social learning, 138
social norms, ix, 142, 151, 152
socioeconomic, 26, 70, 100
socioeconomic status, 26, 70
sodium, 70
spectrum, 97, 100, 102
speed, 92
sperm, 47, 50, 52, 69, 83, 86
spina bifida, 86
spirometry, 114
spontaneous abortion, 48, 52, 53, 71, 74, 77, 87
sporadic, 48
sports, 16
spouse, 49
stages, 112
standard deviation, 93
standard error, 24, 99
standards, 144, 145
state laws, 141
statistics, 80
strategies, 74, 98, 138, 139, 144, 154
strength, 54, 109, 130
stress, 92
structural changes, 92, 94
students, 142
substance use, 64
success rate, 51
sudden infant death syndrome, vii, 1, 3, 8, 11, 47, 58, 72, 74, 80, 82, 93, 121, 123, 152
suppression, 94, 119
surgery, 39, 104, 119, 124
surveillance, 153
susceptibility, 48, 56, 63, 65, 79, 92, 95, 100, 102, 112, 115, 118
symptoms, vii, 1, 3, 8, 11, 39, 76, 97, 101, 105, 106, 107, 108, 110, 112, 118, 120, 152
syndrome, vii, 1, 3, 8, 11, 47, 58, 72, 74, 75, 80, 82, 93, 121, 123, 152
synthesis, 10, 94, 99, 114

systems, vii, 3, 29, 48, 65, 154

T

tandem mass spectrometry, 145
teens, 3
telephone, 28, 51, 105, 133, 136, 140
temporal, 103, 108, 115
teratogenic, 62, 64, 65
theory, 138
therapy, 87
threat, 155
threshold, 123, 144, 152
throat, 104
time periods, 18, 64
timing, 64, 92, 99
tissue, 93
title, 46, 102
tobacco smoking, 7
tonsillectomy, 105, 116
toxic, 52, 114
toxic effect, 114
toxicology, 7
toxin, 97
toxins, 10, 97, 114
transfer, 50, 76, 77, 78
transforming growth factor, 78
transportation, 16, 151
trend, 17, 29, 50, 107
trial, 37, 136, 137, 138, 146, 147
triggers, 118
tumor, 68, 75
tumors, 68, 69, 70, 71, 73, 78, 82

U

ubiquitous, 96
umbilical artery, 75
umbilical cord, 61, 68, 78
umbilical cord blood, 68, 78
uncertainty, 100
underlying mechanisms, 59
underreported, 52
uniform, 29

univariate, 97
urinary, 137
urine, 69, 78
uterus, 69, 83

V

values, 17, 31, 32, 33, 99
vapor, 39
variability, 33, 120
variable, 118
variables, 74, 99, 100, 103
variance, 136
variation, 101
vasoconstriction, 60
vehicles, 2, 23, 35, 136
velocity, 75
ventilation, 33, 144
venue, 145
vessels, 78
viral infection, 100, 102, 109
virus, 122
virus infection, 122
viruses, 102

W

warrants, 54

weight reduction, 62
well-being, 7, 154
western countries, 98
wheeze, 97, 100, 101, 102, 106, 107, 108, 109, 110, 111, 116, 117, 118, 125
wheezing, 110, 120, 123, 126, 127, 128
windows, 48
wives, 53, 79
women, 9, 25, 29, 30, 31, 34, 40, 49, 50, 51, 52, 53, 59, 60, 61, 68, 74, 78, 79, 81, 82, 87, 91, 104, 107, 131, 144, 145, 149, 154
workers, 36, 38, 40, 42, 43, 77, 78, 143, 145, 147
working women, 74
workplace, 15, 23, 25, 32, 33, 34, 35, 38, 39, 42, 47, 48, 53, 81, 124, 139, 140, 143, 145, 146, 149, 151

X

x-rays, 70

Y

young women, 68
younger children, 28, 133